# A COURSE IN MEDICAL AND TECHNICAL TERMINOLOGY

**Joseph R. Tebben**
**Associate Professor of Classics**
**The Ohio State University**

BURGESS INTERNATIONAL GROUP INC
Bellwether Press Division

ISBN 0-8087-2078-3



Printed in the United States of America.
R Q P
Address orders to:

Burgess International Group, Inc.
7110 Ohms Lane
Edina, MN 55435
Telephone 612/831-1344
Telex 29-0458

Bellwether Press
A Division of Burgess International Group, Inc.

# TABLE OF CONTENTS

# ILLUSTRATIONS

# PREFACE

This text is an extension of a course in medical terminology taught by computer instruction at the Ohio State University. It includes all elements and meanings which students are expected to know during their interactive sessions with the computer. This companion text contains a limited number of meanings and variant spellings for the Greek and Latin elements so as to accommodate all possible student responses and to provide diagnostic assistance to correct any student errors in the computer phase of the course. The elements and meanings introduced in each chapter are, therefore, the basic and most generally useful items, but certainly are not exhaustive. This text is in no way a substitute for the manuals of the fields from which the terminology has been drawn and it does not function as a replacement for medical and other specialized dictionaries. The meanings given to the elements are not necessarily their Latin and Greek denotations, but are the meanings which are consistently attached to these forms in the specialized vocabularies of medical and scientific fields.

A guide to pronunciation is provided for each form as it is introduced. The pronunciations are intended to suggest the most commonly heard versions of these forms, but adjustments in these pronunciations will be required for some dialects and in some of the terms employing these components. A medical dictionary with some apparatus for pronunciation is recommended for additional guidance in pronunciation as well as for expansion of the limited materials given in each chapter.

Greek elements have not been separated from Latin elements except in Chapter 15, Numbers, where the distinction is important. The non-philological nature of the students for whom this text is intended and the increasing number of hybrid forms appearing in most dictionaries make the separation of Greek from Latin unnecessary.

Since this text was designed for use in connection with computer instruction, and since the drills and exercises are accomplished by students on computer terminals, only brief exercises are included within the chapters. Two review areas are provided after Chapter 9 and after Chapter 18. These reviews are intended to allow students to check their progress through each half of the course. The discussions and guidelines of the text, however, are generally applicable to all forms of instruction and will serve most students in their understanding of the terminology of medicine and science.

# Chapter 1 55

# INTRODUCTION

Historically the Greek and Latin languages have served as the vehicles of communication in science and medicine. The specialized vocabularies developed from these languages are commonly understood by all speech communities and their classical bases guarantee precision and consistency. While the terminology of scientific fields appears to be complex and difficult to those unfamiliar with Greek and Latin, the terms themselves are composed of simple and recurrent components. The meaning of any technical term can be derived by recognizing the meanings of the individual components and by understanding the principles which govern the arrangement of these components.

There are five types of elements which are used repeatedly in composing technical vocabularies. Each type has a specific function which must be recognized in analyzing a term for its meaning. The first type is called a prefix. A prefix is most often the first component of a technical term and is used to modify the remainder of the term by specifying its intensity, degree, or location. In this way prefixes reflect their original status as Greek and Latin prepositions. Normally only one prefix occurs in each term and it is attached directly to a base form or termination. Hypogeusia, referring to a deficient sense of taste, is composed of the prefix *hypo-* 'deficient' and the termination *-geusia* 'taste'. Hypoglossal, referring to a location below the tongue, is composed of the same prefix *hypo-* 'below', the base form *gloss-* 'tongue', and the suffix *-al* 'pertaining to'. Occasionally several prefixes appear at the beginning of a term. In the term asynchronous, referring to events not occurring together in time, the prefixes *a-* 'not' and *syn-* 'together' are used with the base form *chron-* 'time' and the suffix *-ous* 'pertaining to'. It is also possible to find a prefix embedded in a term to qualify one particular component of the term. The term osteodystrophy, poor development of bones, uses the prefix *dys-* 'poor' after the base form *oste-* 'bone' and before the termination *-trophy* 'development'.

The second type of element is called a base form. A base form is the root (or stem) of a Greek or Latin word and is the major carrier of meaning in a term. Most items in technical vocabularies are base forms. Every term has at least one base form and possibly several of them. In the term neuritis, inflammation of nerves, there is one base form (*neur-* 'nerve') and one suffix (*-itis* 'inflammation').

The third type of element is a combining vowel. Originally a combining vowel (or stem-formative vowel) was used in Greek and Latin to connect the root of the word to its inflectional ending. It is used in terminology to avoid an unpronounceable cluster of consonants or to facilitate pronunciation whenever one base form is added to another element which begins with a consonant. Normally the combining vowel is o, but occasionally other vowels (a, i, y, e, u) are used. When a base form requires a combining vowel other than o it will be indicated in parentheses with the base form. If no combining vowel is indicated with a base form, then o should be used. In the term hepatotomy, incision of the liver, the base form *hepat-* 'liver' is attached to the termination *-tomy* 'incision' by using the combining vowel *-o-*. A combining vowel has no meaning and does not affect the meaning of the term in any way. Since its only function is to ease pronunciation it should not be used unnecessarily. When one base form is added to another element which begins with a vowel there is no need for a combining vowel. When the base form *hepat-* 'liver' is added to the termination *-itis* 'inflammation' no combining vowel is required to produce the term hepatitis. It is possible to have as many combining vowels in a term as there are base forms, but each combining vowel must be justified by having the successive base form begin with a consonant. Because combining vowels are so common, occasionally terms are found which use a combining vowel where none is required. This unnecessary use of combining vowels has resulted from analogy with the many instances where combining vowels are needed. Nevertheless, the use of unnecessary combining vowels should be avoided when terms are formulated from definitions.

The suffix is the fourth type of element. A suffix is always the last component of a term and specifies the essential meaning of the term as well as its grammatical function. Only noun-forming, verb-forming, and adjective-forming suffixes are presented in this text. In a few instances two suffixes may occur in one term, but usually each term has only one suffix as its final element. In the adjective gastric, the base form *gastr-* 'stomach' is added to the suffix *-ic* 'pertaining to'.

The fifth type of element, the termination, is actually a combination of a base form and a suffix, or a prefix, base form, and suffix. Since selected elements tend to occur so frequently together they are considered to be a unit and an all inclusive meaning is assigned to the termination. The several elements used to compose each termination are shown in parentheses beneath the termination as it is listed in the text. The term splenectopy, displacement of the spleen, is formed from the base form *splen-* 'spleen' and the termination *-ectopy* 'displacement'. The termination itself contains the prefix *ec-* 'out', the base form *top-* 'place', and the suffix *-y* 'state of'.

When the meanings of these basic elements are understood, the full meaning of any technical term can be obtained by analyzing the ordering of these elements. Each term imparts meaning at several levels. The first level of meaning is given by the final element of the term, the suffix or termination. At this level the term is given its essential meaning and its grammatical function. In the term gastradenitis, the suffix *-itis* provides the basic meaning of 'inflammation' and indicates that the term is a noun. Each additional level gives more specific information about the basic meaning of the suffix or termination. Gastradenitis uses the base form *aden-* 'gland' to modify the suffix *-itis* and gives the meaning 'inflammation of glands'. Any level may further refine the meaning of the elements following it. In the term gastradenitis, the last level *gastr-* 'stomach' specifies the location of the inflamed glands. The full definition of the term gastradenitis by levels is 'inflammation of the glands of the stomach'. Each of the levels which makes the term more specific is called subordinating. It is also possible for any level to provide information which parallels the information of the preceding level. Since a level of this sort does not refine the meaning of the previous levels but is of equal importance it is called coordinating. In the term gastrocolitis, the inflammation (*-itis*) is located in the stomach (*gastr-*) and the colon (*col-*). Coordinating levels are recognized in a definition by the word 'and' since neither level is subordinate to the other. The location of coordinating elements within a term and its definition is to some extent arbitrary. The definition of gastrocolitis is 'inflammation of the stomach and colon' or 'inflammation of the colon and stomach'.

Both coordinating and subordinating levels can be found within a term and the number of levels can be repeated indefinitely. Most technical terms contain three or four elements. The levels of several medical terms are graphically indicated below.

**gastroscopy**

gastr-o- -scopy

examination

of the stomach

**dermatomycosis**

dermat-o- myc- -osis

abnormal condition

of fungus

of the skin

**psychosomatic**

psych-o- somat- -ic

pertaining to

the mind and the body

The meaning of any term is usually obtained by proceeding from the last part of the term to the first part. The only exception involves coordinating levels where the direction may be arbitrary. This process is reversed when terms are to be created from definitions. The first item of the definition is the suffix or termination, the last element of the term, and the remaining parts of the definition become the elements which precede the suffix or termination in either coordinating or subordinating levels. 'Excision of stones from the bladder' by levels is

excision

-ectomy

of stones

lith-

from the bladder

cyst-o-

and produces the term cystolithectomy. 'The study of the stomach and small intestines' by levels is

study

-logy

of the stomach and small intestines

gastr-o- enter-o-

and the term gastroenterology results. Notice the analogous use of the combining vowel with gastr- and the necessary use of the combining vowel before -logy.

Each chapter of the text contains a list of prefixes, base forms, suffixes, and terminations. All forms are listed with hyphens to indicate their incomplete status and their relative position when used to construct larger forms. While some of these forms do exist independently (e.g. lymph) or with the addition of simple noun-forming suffixes like -a and -ma (e.g. plasma, cornea), in this text they will be used as components of larger forms. Many base forms have alternate spellings because of variation in the stem of the original Greek or Latin word. The most frequently used spelling is given first. Other important alternate spellings of the same form follow. Occasionally two distinct base forms are given with the same meaning. This occurs whenever Greek synonymous forms have been incorporated into technical terminology, or whenever both the Greek and Latin words for the same item are used. Some of these base forms are marked with an asterisk to show that they are used infrequently to construct terms. Recognition of these infrequently used forms is important, but the more frequently used base forms should be employed to construct terms from definitions.

Prefixes never use combining vowels. Since most prefixes end in a vowel, they are attached directly to a base form beginning with a consonant. Whenever the base form to which a prefix is to be attached begins with a vowel the final vowel of the prefix is usually deleted. The prefix *endo-* is directly attached to the consonant-initial base form *derm-* to form endodermal. The same prefix becomes *end-* when added to the vowel-initial base form *odont-* to form endodontitis. Prefixes are listed in their full form, without notice of the possible elimination of the final vowel.

Information supplied in parentheses about the meaning of an element is not part of the meaning of the element but is given to facilitate understanding of the element as it is used in technical terminology. One of the most troublesome matters in creating terms to match definitions is the selection of the correct element from among several elements which have the same meaning. Several suffixes, for example, mean 'pertaining to'. To some degree the preference of one such suffix over another is determined by the Latin or Greek status of the form to which a suffix must be added. The Greek base form *derm-* accepts the suffix *-ic* in the term hypodermic. In other instances, however, the Latin suffix *-al* is used with the Greek *derm-*, as in epidermal. The context sensitivity which allows some formulations of elements and rejects other theoretically possible combinations can best be acquired by exposure to the terminology as it actually exists. When there is doubt about the validity of a formulation, a medical dictionary should be consulted.

A pronunciation is provided for each element as it is introduced. The pronunciation approximates the sounds of the elements as they are used in many vocabulary items. Obviously the pronunciation must be adjusted where specific terms require modification. Most consonant sounds are consistent and obvious. The letter g is pronounced [j] before e, i, y; otherwise it is to be pronounced as [g]. The letter c before e, i, y is pronounced [s]; elsewhere it is pronounced [k]. [ŋ] represents the final nasal sound in the word ring. Forms which begin with two consonants unblended in English (pm, ps, pt, gn) sound only the second of these consonants when the form is used initially. If the consonant clusters are preceded by vowels, however, both consonants are usually sounded but in different syllables. Consonants which belong to the preceding or following syllable will be marked in the pronunciation guide by a raised dot. The vowel scheme used in the pronunciation guide is

| vowel sound | as in |
|---|---|
| [ā] | bait |
| [a] | bat |
| [ä] | bar |
| [ē] | beet |
| [e] | bet |
| [ə] | but |
| [ī] | bite |
| [i] | bit |
| [ō] | boat |
| [o] | born |
| [ū] | boot |
| [yū] | beaut(y) |
| [u] | bull |
| [aw] | bout |
| [oy] | boil |

In the examples given in the text the primary accent (stress) for each word is indicated by ' preceding the syllable to be accented (stressed).

| Elements | Pronunciations | Meanings | Examples |
|---|---|---|---|
| *Prefixes* | | | |
| hyper- | [hīpər] | excessive | hyper'pnea |
| hypo- | [hīpō] | deficient, below | hypo'tonia |
| ec-, ex-(before vowels) | [ek] | out | ec'topic |
| ecto-, exo- | [ektō] | outer, outside | ecto'cytic |
| endo-, ento- | [endō] | inner, inside, within | endorhi'nitis |
| tele | [telɔ] | at a distance, afar | tele'cardiogram |
| *Base Forms* | | | |
| anthrop- | [anthrōp] | man, human being | 'misanthrope |
| bi- | [bī, bē] | life, living | symbi'osis |
| chron- | [krän] | time | chro'nology |
| cicatric- | [sikətrik] | scar | cicatri'cotomy |

| Elements | Pronunciations | Meanings | Examples |
|---|---|---|---|
| dem- | [dem] | people, country | en'demic |
| dermat-, derm- | [dərmət] | skin | derma'tologist |
| eti- | [ētē] | cause | eti'ology |
| ge- | [jē] | earth | ge'ologist |
| hypn- | [hip·n] | sleep | hyp'notic |
| iatr- | [īə·tr] | healing | ia'trology |
| kym- | [kīm] | wave | 'kymogram |
| log- | [log, ləj] | word, understanding | ne'ologist |
| nyct- | [nikt] | night | nyctambly'opia |
| od-, hod- | [ōd] | road, way | 'cathode |
| ped- | [pēd] | child | pedo'dontics |
| pharmac- | [färmək] | drug | 'pharmacist |
| phon- | [fōn, fän] | sound, voice | 'phonic |
| psych- | [sīk] | mind, soul | psychoso'matic |
| squam- | [skwäm] | scale, flake | 'desquamate |
| therm- | [thərm] | heat | 'diathermy |
| ton- | [tōn, tän] | tension | to'nometry |
| top- | [tōp, täp] | place | topes'thesia |
| all- | [al] | other, different | allo'morphic |
| atel- | [atel] | incomplete, imperfect | atelo'cardia |
| aut- | [awt] | self, one's own | au'togenous |
| eur(y)- | [yur] | wide | eu'ryphagous |
| megal-, meg(a)- | [megəl] | large | megalo'karyocyte |
| pant- | [pant] | all, complete | 'pantograph |
| pseud | [sūd] | false | pseudocy'esis |
| sten- | [sten] | narrow | steno'cardia |

*Suffixes*

| | | | |
|---|---|---|---|
| -ia | [ēə] | condition of | di'coria |
| -sis, -sia | [sis, sēə] | condition of | 'synthesis |
| -y | [ē] | state of | cardio'megaly |
| -al | [əl] | pertaining to | 'dermal |

| Elements | Pronunciations | Meanings | Examples |
|---|---|---|---|
| -ic | [ic] | pertaining to | ana'crotic |
| -ate | [āt] | to make | 'phonate |
| -ize | [īz] | to make | 'synchronize |

*Terminations*

| Elements | Pronunciations | Meanings | Examples |
|---|---|---|---|
| -itis | [ītis] | inflammation | derma'titis |
| -osis | [ōsis] | abnormal condition | throm'bosis |
| -ist | [ist] | one who (specializes in) | radi'ologist |
| -scope (scop/e) | [skōp] | instrument for examining | sig'moidoscope |
| -scopy (scop/y) | [skəpē] | examination | sigmoi'doscopy |
| -gram | [gram] | a record(ing) | electro'cardiogram |
| -graphy (graph/y) | [grafē] | state of recording | cardi'ography |
| -algia (alg/ia) | [aljēə] | pain | cephal'algia |
| -ectomy (ec/tom/y) | [ektōmē] | excision, surgical removal | appen'dectomy |
| -stenosis (sten/o/sis) | [stenōsis] | narrowing | gastrosten'osis |
| -logy (log/y) | [ləjē] | study | laryn'gology |
| -ics (ic/s) | [iks] | system | 'optics |

Two very common terminations in the language of medicine are -itis and -osis. Originally the element -itis formed a feminine adjective which was then used to qualify the Greek word for disease, *nosos*. The Greek *arthritis nosos* was used to identify a disease pertaining to the joints. Since the disease referred to so often was inflammation, gradually the word for disease was dropped and the adjective-forming element -itis acquired the meaning inflammation. The termination -osis is, strictly speaking, a combination of the combining vowel -o- and the noun-forming suffix -sis. The suffix has the meaning of condition, but since so often in medicine the condition is abnormal it has been found useful to apply the meaning 'abnormal condition' to the termination -osis.

*Exercise*

Complete the terms below by using the definitions on the right.

| | | |
|---|---|---|
| 1. | ( auto )nomous | self regulating |
| 2. | (megalo )cardia | a condition of a large heart |
| 3. | (pseud )onym | a false name |
| 4. | ( endo )tracheal | within the trachea |
| 5. | (chrono )meter | an instrument to measure time |
| 6. | sigmoido(scope ) | an instrument for examining the sigmoid flexure |
| 7. | tonsill(ectomy ) | excision of the tonsils |
| 8. | entero(stenosis ) | narrowing of the small intestine |
| 9. | ( atelo )myelia | condition of an incomplete spinal cord |
| 10. | ( ped )iatric | pertaining to the healing of children |

Provide definitions for the following terms.

1. anthropology ___ study of man ___
2. dermatitis ___ inflammation of the skin ___
3. hypothermia ___ cond. of deficient heat ___
4. hypodermic ___ pertaining to below the skin ___
5. phonologist ______
6. pharmacist ______
7. autobiography ______
8. etiology ______
9. nyctalgia ______
10. hypogeal ______

# Chapter 2 (59)

# GENERAL MATERIALS

| Elements | Pronunciations | Meanings | Examples |
|---|---|---|---|
| *Prefixes* | | | |
| super- | [sūpər] | over, excessive | superlac'tation |
| supra- | [sūprə] | above | supra'pubic |
| pro- | [prō] | forward | 'prodrome |
| pan- | [pan] | all, complete | panophthal'mitis |
| para- | [parə] | beside, abnormal | para'sternal |
| *Base Forms* | | | |
| actin- | [aktin] | ray, x ray | actinoneu'ritis |
| adenoid- | [adinoyd] | adenoid | adenoid'ectomy |
| bar- | [bar] | weight, pressure | bares'thesia |
| chromat-, chrom- | [krōmət] | color | chromat'osis |
| drom- | [drōm] | running, course | 'syndrome |
| dyn-, dynam- | [dīnəm] | power | dyna'mometer |
| electr- | [əlek·tr] | electricity | electrodyna'mometer |
| heli- | [hēlē] | sun | helio'therapy |
| my- | [mī] | muscle | myomela'nosis |
| phot- | [fōt] | light | photoderma'titis |
| radi- | [rādē] | ray, x ray | radiopath'ology |
| radic-, radicul- | [radik] | root | radi'cotomy |
| rhiz- | [rīz] | root | 'rhizoid |
| somat-, som- | [sōmat] | body | somato'pathic |
| tonsill- | [tänsil] | tonsil | tonsill'ectomy |
| tox-, tox(i)- | [toks] | poison | tox'iferous |
| bar(y)- | [bar] | heavy | bary'glossia |

| Elements | Pronunciations | Meanings | Examples |
|---|---|---|---|
| brad(y)- | [brad] | slow | bradyp'nea |
| dextr- | [dek·str] | right | dextro'gastria |
| dist- | [dist] | farthest | 'distal |
| heter- | [hetər] | other, different | heterochroma'tosis |
| hom- | [hōm] | same | homo'chronous |
| home- | [hōmē] | similar | homeo'morphous |
| is- | [īs] | equal | 'isobar |
| lei- | [lī] | smooth | lei'otrichous |
| lept- | [lept] | thin, delicate | 'leptosome |
| medi- | [mēdē] | middle | medio'tarsal |
| mes-, mesi- | [mez] | middle | meso'philic |
| ne- | [nē] | new | neo'plasia |
| pach(y)- | [pak] | thick | pachy'dermatous |
| proxim- | [präksim] | nearest | 'proximate |
| sinistr- | [sinis·tr] | left | sinistro'cardia |
| tach(y)- | [tak] | rapid, fast | tachy'phagia |
| trach(y)- | [trāk, trak] | rough | trach'oma |
| crin- | [krin] | secrete | crino'genic |
| pha-, phas-, phem- | [fā, fāz, fēm] | speak | dys'phasia |
| phag- | [fag] | eat, swallow | phagocy'tolysis |

*Suffixes*

| | | | |
|---|---|---|---|
| -e | | instrument | 'gastrotome |
| -t | | instrument | 'osteoclast |

Both of these suffixes may be used to form nouns without adding the meaning 'instrument'. Such is the case in terms like chromosome and leukocyte.

| | | | |
|---|---|---|---|
| -oid | [oyd] | resembling, like | 'toxoid |
| -ary | [erē] | pertaining to | 'sanguinary |
| -ous | [us] | pertaining to | a'chromatous |
| -tic | [tik] | pertaining to | cata'lytic |

The adjectival suffix -tic is used to convert nouns ending in -sis and -sia into adjectives. The noun hematolysis becomes the adjective hematolytic when this suffix is applied.

| Elements | Pronunciations | Meanings | Examples |
|---|---|---|---|
| *Terminations* | | | |
| -meter | [mətər] | instrument to measure | sphyg'mometer |
| -metry (metr/y) | [mətrē] | measurement | te'lemetry |
| -tome (tom/e) | [tōm] | instrument to cut | 'gastrotome |
| -tomy (tom/y) | [tōmē] | incision | gas'trotomy |
| -ectasis, -ectasia (ec/ta/sis) | [ektāzēə] | dilatation, stretching | enterec'tasia |
| -ectopy, -ectopia (ec/top/y) | [ektəpē] | displacement | my'ectopy |
| -odynia (odyn/ia) | [ōdinēə] | pain | dorso'dynia |
| -malacia (malac/ia) | [məlāshə] | softening | osteoma'lacia |
| -esthesia (esthe/sia) | [esthēzēə] | sensitivity, perception | pares'thesia |
| -geusia (geu/sia) | [gyūzeə] | taste | para'geusia |
| -lysis (ly/sis) | [lisis] | dissolution, destruction | li'tholysis |
| -ician (ic/ian) | [ishən] | specialist in | op'tician |

The element adenoid- is composed of the suffix -oid (from the Greek word *eidos* meaning form or shape) and the Greek word *aden* meaning acorn. Thus the adenoids are named from their appearance as acorn-like. The Greek element for muscle, my-, also is the Greek word for mouse. The movement of muscles beneath the skin suggested the passage of little mice. Indeed, the English word muscle is derived from the Latin *musculus,* meaning little mouse. The element tox- is derived from the Greek word for bow. It has acquired the meaning of poison from the practice of putting poisons on the tips of arrows as they were launched from bows at enemies. And the element electr- originally referred to amber. Because amber was so easily charged by friction the Greek word *electron* became associated with electricity.

*Exercise*

Complete the terms below by using the definitions on the right.

1. (brady)pepsia — slow digestion
2. (helio)tropic — turning toward the sun
3. (supra)renal — above the kidney
4. (radio therapist — one who gives x ray treatments
5. cyt(oid) — resembling a cell
6. a(phas)ia — a condition of not speaking (properly)
7. cranio(malacia) — softening of the skull
8. osteo(tome) — an instrument to cut bone
9. (hetero)morphic — pertaining to a different form
10. hemato(lysis) — destruction of blood

Provide definitions for the following terms.

1. myodynamia cond. of powerful muscles
2. toxic pert. to poison
3. photometer inst. to measure light
4. actinodermitis infl. of skin due to x-rays
5. panchromatic pert. to all colors
6. paraphemia cond. of abnormal speech
7. eurysomic pertain. to wide body
8. electrolysis dissolution due to electricity
9. rhizotomy incision of roots
10. pandemic pert. to all the countrys/people

# Chapter 3

# SUBSTANCES, FLUIDS

Prefixes which end in a consonant often appear in modified forms in terminology. These modifications result from a linguistic process called assimilation (or morphophonemic change) which changes the final consonant of the prefix to facilitate its pronunciation before elements beginning with certain consonants. Generally the final consonant of the prefix is altered so that it more closely resembles the class of sound to which the initial consonant of the base form belongs. The final consonant of the prefix can become more like, but not identical with, the initial consonant of the base form by partial assimilation. The prefix *syn-* appears as *sym-* when it is attached to base forms beginning with p, b, or ph. Thus the prefix *syn-* becomes *sym-* in the terms sympodia, symbiosis, and symphysis. When the final consonant of the prefix becomes identical with the initial consonant of the base form total assimilation has occurred. The prefix *con-* before base forms beginning with l or r becomes *col-* in collateral and *cor-* in corrugator. Total assimilation almost always occurs with the prefixes *ad-* and *sub-*. The terms appendix (ad—pendix), afferent (ad—ferent) and suppression (sub—pression) display total assimilation. Assimilation never occurs with the Latin prefix *a-, ab-, abs-* 'away from, from'. Occasionally the final consonant of a prefix is eliminated when the prefix is added to a base form beginning with two or more consonants. The term systole is composed of the prefix *syn-* and the termination *-stole.*

Prefixes ending in a consonant are listed first in their non-assimilated form. This form of the prefix is used before vowels and most consonants. The major assimilated forms of the prefix are listed after the more usual form.

| Elements | Pronunciations | Meanings | Examples |
|---|---|---|---|
| *Prefixes* | | | |
| ad- | [ad] | to, toward, near | ad'neural |
| a-, ab-, abs- | [ab] | away from, from | abar'ticular |
| en-, em-, el- | [en] | in, into | 'enthesis |
| sub-, suc-, suf- | [səb] | under | sub'lingual |
| *Base Forms* | | | |
| aur-, aur(i)- | [awr] | gold | 'auric |
| chrys- | [kris] | gold | chryso'therapy |
| argent(i)-, argent- | [ärjent] | silver | ar'gentous |

| Elements | Pronunciations | Meanings | Examples |
|---|---|---|---|
| ferr(i)-, ferr- | [fer] | iron | fer'rometer |
| corn(i)-, corn(u)- | [korn] | horn | cor'niculate |
| kerat- | [kerət] | horn | keratoderma'titis |
| lith- | [lith] | stone, calculus | lith'uria |
| hal(i)-, hal- | [hal] | salt | 'halogen |
| sal(i)- | [sal] | salt | sa'limeter |
| hyal- | [hīəl] | glass | 'hyaloid |
| vitr-, vitr(i)- | [vi·tr] | glass | 'vitriform |
| glyc-, gluc- | [glīk, glūk] | sugar | gly'colysis |
| sacchar- | [sakər] | sugar | saccharo'lytic |
| myc-, mycet- | [mīk, mīset] | fungus | actinomy'cosis |
| seb-, seb(i)- | [seb] | tallow, grease | 'sebolith |
| steat-, stear- | [stēät, stēär] | tallow | ste'atocele |
| adip- | [adip] | (animal) fat | 'adipoid |
| lip- | [lip] | fat | 'lipocele |
| amyl- | [amil] | starch | 'amylase |
| coll- | [kol] | glue, gelatin | coll'oma |
| blenn- | [blen] | mucus | blenno'stasis |
| muc-, muc(i)- | [myūk] | mucus, mucous membrane | mucoente'ritis |
| myx- | [miks] | mucus | myxo'rrhea |
| py- | [pī] | pus | pyarth'rosis |
| ptyal- | [tīəl] | saliva | pty'alagogue |
| sial- | [sīəl] | saliva | sialoli'thiasis |
| ole- | [ōlē] | oil | o'leic |
| acet-, acet(i)- | [əsēt] | acid, vinegar | a'cetify |
| hydr- | [hī·dr] | water, fluid | hydro'therapy |
| *aqu(e)-, aqu(a)- | [ā·kw] | water | 'aqueous |
| hygr- | [hī·gr] | moisture | hy'grometer |
| hidr- | [hī·dr] | sweat | hyperhi'drosis |
| galact- | [galakt] | milk | galacto'rrhea |
| lact-, lact(i)- | [lakt] | milk | lacto'genic |
| pyr-, pyret- | [pīrət] | fire, fever | pyreto'genic |

| Elements | Pronunciations | Meanings | Examples |
|---|---|---|---|
| *Suffixes* | | | |
| -in, -ine | [in, ēn] | substance | 'toxin |
| -ase | [ās, āz] | enzyme | 'lipase |
| -ate | [āt] | having | 'dentate |
| -ose | [ōs] | full of, pertaining to | 'foliose |
| -ad | [ad] | toward, in the direction of | 'mesiad |
| -eal | [ēəl] | pertaining to | pha'ryngeal |

The adjective-forming suffix *-eal* is used especially when the preceding element ends in the letter g.

| Elements | Pronunciations | Meanings | Examples |
|---|---|---|---|
| -fy | [fī] | to make | 'ramify |
| *Terminations* | | | |
| -agogue | [əgog] | agent inducing flow | si'alagogue |
| -form | [form] | having the shape of | 'vermiform |
| -oma | [ōmə] | tumor | myx'oma |
| -omatous (omat/ous) | [ōmətus] | pertaining to tumors | myx'omatous |
| -omatosis (omat/o/sis) | [ōmətōsis] | abnormal condition of tumors | myxoma'tosis |
| -ferous, -feric (fer/ous) | [fərus] | bearing, carrying | lac'tiferous |
| -genous, -genic (gen/ic) | [jenik] | causing, caused by | carcino'genic |
| -therapy (therap/y) | [therəpē] | treatment | auro'therapy |
| -rrhea (rrhe/a) | [rēə] | flow | meno'rrhea |
| -poiesis (poie/sis) | [poyēsis] | production, formation | cholepoi'esis |

The termination -oma is composed of the combining vowel -o- and the Greek noun-forming suffix -ma. It has acquired the specialized meaning of tumor from its use in the term carcinoma, used by the Greeks to describe a creeping ulcer or eating sore. The term itself is formed from the Greek word for crab, *carcinos,* either because the ulcer spread crab-wise or because the veins in the area affected resembled the shape of crab claws. The English word cancer is borrowed from the Latin *cancer* meaning both crab and creeping ulcer. The element -therapy is based upon the Greek word for attendant or servant, *therapon.*

*Exercise*

Complete the terms below by using the definitions at the right.

| | |
|---|---|
| 1. ( amyl )emia | the presence of starch in the blood |
| 2. ( hydro )cephalic | pertaining to fluid in the head |
| 3. anti( pyret )ic | pertaining to (an agent acting) against fever |
| 4. ( hal / sal )oid | resembling salt |
| 5. ( myco )myring( itis ) | fungus inflammation of the tympanic membrane |
| 6. ( lact / galact )in | a milk substance |
| 7. ( pyo )cele | a swelling (containing) pus |
| 8. cephal( ad ) | toward the head |
| 9. chole( poiesis ) | formation of bile |
| 10. blenno( rrhea ) | flow of mucus |

Provide definitions for the following terms.

1. adipoma tumor of (animal) fat
2. aurotherapy treatment w/ gold
3. hidradenitis inflammation of sweat gland
4. seborrhea flow of grease (tallow)
5. hygroscope inst. for exam. moisture
6. lactagogue agent ind. flow of milk
7. toxiferous carrying poison
8. keratin horn substance
9. hypoliposis abn. cond. of deficient fat
10. mycology study of fungus

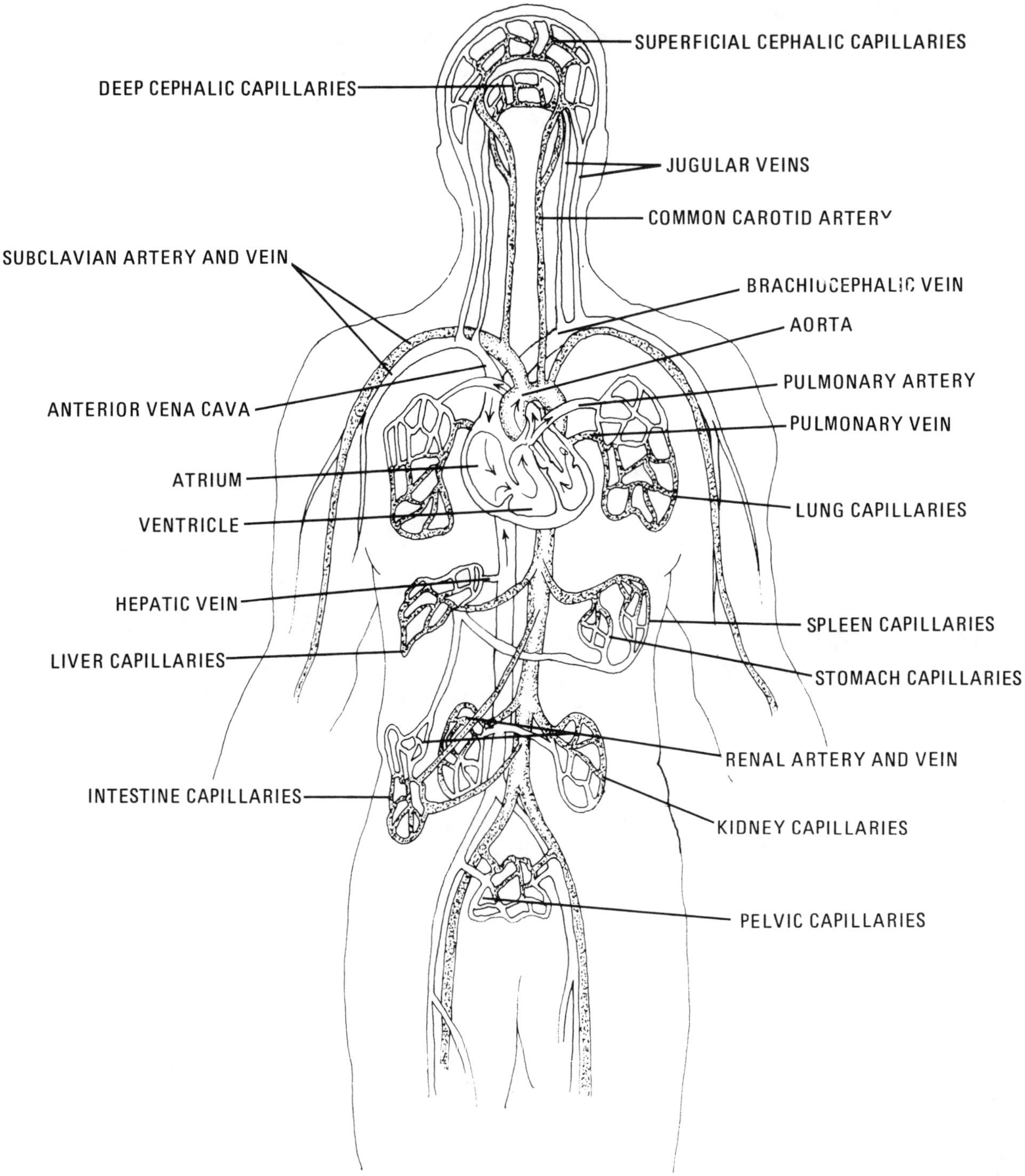
SUPERFICIAL CEPHALIC CAPILLARIES
DEEP CEPHALIC CAPILLARIES
JUGULAR VEINS
COMMON CAROTID ARTERY
SUBCLAVIAN ARTERY AND VEIN
BRACHIOCEPHALIC VEIN
AORTA
PULMONARY ARTERY
ANTERIOR VENA CAVA
PULMONARY VEIN
ATRIUM
LUNG CAPILLARIES
VENTRICLE
HEPATIC VEIN
SPLEEN CAPILLARIES
LIVER CAPILLARIES
STOMACH CAPILLARIES
RENAL ARTERY AND VEIN
INTESTINE CAPILLARIES
KIDNEY CAPILLARIES
PELVIC CAPILLARIES

**PLATE I**

# Chapter 4

# CIRCULATORY SYSTEM

| Elements | Pronunciations | Meanings | Examples |
|---|---|---|---|
| *Prefixes* | | | |
| anti- | [antē] | against | anti'toxin |
| dys- | [dis] | poor, painful | dys'chezia |
| a-, an- | [ā, an] | not, without | a'thrombia |

The most common negative prefix in medical terminology is *a-, an-*. It appears as *an-* before elements beginning with vowels or the letter h (an—esthesia, an—hydrous), as *a-* before elements beginning with consonants.

| Elements | Pronunciations | Meanings | Examples |
|---|---|---|---|
| *Base Forms* | | | |
| cardi- | [kärdē] | heart | 'cardiocele |
| atri- | [ātrē] | atrium | 'atriotome |
| *auricul- | [orikyūl] | auricle, atrium | auriculoven'tricular |
| ventricul- | [ventrikyūl] | ventricle | ven'tricular |
| aort- | [āort] | aorta | aortoma'lacia |
| arteri- | [ärtērē] | artery | arterioste'nosis |
| capillar- | [kapilər] | capillary | capilla'ritis |
| phleb- | [fleb] | vein | phle'bitis |
| *ven- | [vēn] | vein | 'venogram |
| angi- | [anjē] | vessel | 'angioblast |
| *vascul- | [vaskyūl] | vessel | vascu'litis |
| hem-, hemat- | [hēmət] | blood | hema'toma |
| blast- | [blast] | embryonic cell | 'blastomere |
| kary- | [karē] | nucleus | 'karyophage |
| cyt- | [sīt] | cell | leukocy'temia |
| globul- | [gläbyul] | globule, corpuscle | 'globulism |
| plasm- | [plas·m] | plasma | 'plasmosome |
| ser- | [sir] | serum | se'rologist |

| Elements | Pronunciations | Meanings | Examples |
|---|---|---|---|
| thromb- | [thrämb] | clot | thrombokin'esis |
| puls(i)-, puls- | [puls] | pulse | pul'sation |
| sphygm- | [sfig·m] | pulse | sphygmo'cardiogram |
| crot- | [krät] | pulse beat | di'crotic |
| lymph- | [limf] | lymph | lymphangi'ectasis |
| splen- | [splen] | spleen | sple'nectopy |
| aden- | [adin] | gland | adeno'dynia |
| path- | [path] | disease | pa'thologist |
| phil- | [fil] | love | phil'anthropist |
| phob- | [fōb] | fear | nycto'phobia |
| erythr- | [erith·r] | red | e'rythroblast |
| leuk- | [lūk] | white | leu'kemia |
| cyan- | [sīən] | blue | acrocya'nosis |
| sta- | [sta] | stop, control | 'static |

*Suffix*

| | | | |
|---|---|---|---|
| -ac | [ak] | pertaining to | 'cardiac |

*Terminations*

| | | | |
|---|---|---|---|
| -emia (em/ia) | [ēmēə] | blood condition | ur'emia |
| -blast | [blast] | embryonic cell | 'myeloblast |
| -cyte (cyt/e) | [sīt] | cell | 'macrocyte |
| -lith | [lith] | stone, calculus | 'rhinolith |
| -stasis (sta/sis) | [stəsis, stasis] | stopping, controlling | throm'bostasis |
| -kinesis, -kinesia (kine/sis) | [kinēsis] | movement | dyskin'esis |
| -pathy (path/y) | [pəthē] | a disease | hepa'topathy |
| -philia (phil/ia) | [filēə] | affinity, love | photo'philia |

| Elements | Pronunciations | Meanings | Examples |
|---|---|---|---|
| -sclerosis (scler/o/sis) | [sklərōsis] | hardening | angioscle'rosis |
| -megaly (megal/y) | [megəlē] | enlargement | cardio'megaly |
| -cele (cel/e) | [sēl] | hernia(tion), swelling | en'cephalocele |
| -penia (pen/ia) | [pēnēə] | deficiency | lympho'penia |
| -plegia (pleg/ia) | [plējēə] | paralysis, stroke | hemi'plegia |
| -ptosis (pto/sis) | [p·tōsis] | prolapse, sagging | aortop'tosis |
| -rrhexis (rrhex/is) | [reksis] | rupture | phlebo'rrhexis |
| -sepsis (sep/sis) | [sepsis] | infection | entero'sepsis |
| -centesis (cente/sis) | [sentēsis] | surgical puncture | rachicen'tesis |
| -clysis (cly/sis) | [klisis, klīsis] | irrigation, washing | ve'noclysis |
| -pexy (pex/y) | [peksē] | fixation | 'colopexy |
| -piesis (pie/sis) | [pīēsis] | pressure | hyperpi'esis |
| -plasty (plast/y) | [plastē] | surgical repair | ar'terioplasty |
| -rrhaphy (rrhaph/y) | [rəfē] | suture | cardi'orrhaphy |
| -trophy, -trophia (troph/y) | [trōfē] | development | hy'pertrophy |

Base forms which end in a vowel, like cardi- and arteri- of this chapter, normally drop that final vowel when they are added to a suffix or termination beginning with that same vowel. Arteritis and carditis reflect this simplification of two identical vowels into one. However, when a base form ending in a vowel is to be attached to a base form beginning with that same vowel both vowels are retained and separated by a hyphen. Salpingo-oophorectomy demonstrates this use of the hyphen. On rare occasions a hyphen may even appear between a prefix and a base form, as in extra-articular, but only when the usual deleting of the final vowel fo the prefix does not facilitate pronunciation.

The termination *-emia* of this chapter can be preceded by a base form which indicates the location of the condition or by a base form indicating the presence of foreign matter in the blood. Splenemia means 'blood condition (congestion) of the spleen'. Cholemia means 'a condition of bile in the blood' or 'a blood condition of bile (presence)'.

The two words auricle and ventricle are examples of diminutives, elements which have acquired special suffixes to convey the notion of reduced size. Auricle, literally meaning little ear, is derived from the Latin word for ear, *auris.* The Latin *venter,* stomach or belly, has acquired the diminutive suffix in the term ventricle. Both terms are applied to small chambers in the heart. The capillaries are named after their resemblance to hair, *capillus* being the Latin word for hair.

A common problem developing in the circulatory system is atheroschlerosis. This condition results when the walls of the arteries become thickened because of fatty accumulations within blood vessels. *Athere* is the Greek word for porridge. Another occurrence within the circulatory system is the obstruction of blood vessels by blood clots. This condition is called embolism, a term constructed from the Greek word *ballein,* to throw, and the Greek preposition, *en,* in, which has been assimilated to em-. Finally there is the condition of anemia. Literally this term implies a condition of being without blood, but actually it is a misnomer for a condition of reduced levels of red blood cells or hemoglobin.

*Exercise*

Complete the terms below by using the definitions at the right.

| | |
|---|---|
| 1. (antithromb)in | a substance (acting) against clots |
| 2. osteo(dystrophy) | poor development of the bones |
| 3. (leukocyt)osis | abnormal condition of white (blood) cells |
| 4. (dysphag)ia | a condition of painful swallowing |
| 5. (Karyo)rrhexis | nuclear rupture |
| 6. (lympho)cyto(penia) | deficiency of lymph cells |
| 7. (angio)lith | calculus in a (blood) vessel |
| 8. (hemopatho)logy | study of blood disease |
| 9. angio(rrhapy) | suture of a (blood) vessel |
| 10. (erythrocyt)e | a red (blood) cell |

Provide definitions for the following terms.

1. splenorrhaphy ___ suture of the spleen
2. hypopiesis ___ low (blood) pressure
3. cardiocele ___ swelling of the heart
4. sphygmophone ___ instrument that gives sound to pulses.
5. thrombokinesis ___ movement of clots
6. arteriosclerosis ___ hardening of the arterys
7. angiectasia ___ stretching of vessels
8. serology ___ study of serum
9. hemangioma ___ tumor in a blood vessel
10. splenectomy ___ excision of the spleen

# Chapter 5

# NERVOUS SYSTEM

| Elements | Pronunciations | Meanings | Examples |
|---|---|---|---|
| *Prefixes* | | | |
| ana- | [anə] | up, again | anabi'osis |
| re- | [rē] | back, again | re'vive |
| cata- | [katə] | down, very | cata'tropic |
| de- | [di, dē] | down, away | de'ciduous |
| ante- | [antē, anti] | before, in front | ante'prostate |
| pre- | [prē] | before | pregangli'onic |
| meta- | [metə] | after, changed | meta'tarsal |
| post- | [pōst] | after, behind | postencepha'litis |
| dia- | [dīə] | through, across | diag'nosis |
| trans- | [tranz] | across | trans'septal |
| amphi-, ampho- | [amfi] | both, on both sides | am'phitrichous |
| inter- | [intər] | between, among | inter'crural |
| circum- | [sircum] | around | circum'lental |
| intra-, intro- | [intrə] | within | intra'cystic |
| extra-, extro- | [ekstrə] | outside, beyond | extra-ar'ticular |
| infra- | [infrə] | below | infra'scapular |
| dis-, di-, dif- | [dis] | apart | 'dissect |
| *Base Forms* | | | |
| cephal- | [sefəl] | head | cephalocen'tesis |
| encephal- | [ensefəl] | brain | encephalopy'osis |
| cerebell- | [serəbel] | cerebellum | cerebello'spinal |
| cerebr- | [serə·br] | cerebrum | cerebroscle'rosis |
| neur- | [nūr] | nerve | polyneu'ritis |

| Elements | Pronunciations | Meanings | Examples |
|---|---|---|---|
| gangli-, ganglion- | [gaŋ gli] | ganglion | ganglioneur'oma |
| astr- | [as·tr] | star, star-shaped | 'astrocyte |
| stell- | [stel] | star, star-shaped | 'stellate |
| myel- | [mīəl] | spinal cord | myel'atrophy |
| mening- | [meninj] | meninges | menin'gitis |
| mer- | [mər] | part | mo'nomerous |
| poli- | [pōlī] | gray (matter) | polioencepha'litis |
| micr- | [mī·kr] | small | microg'nathia |
| macr- | [ma·kr] | large | 'macrocyte |
| dolich- | [dolik] | long | dolicho'pelvic |
| brach(y)- | [brak] | short | brachydac'tylia |
| *nerv(i)- | [nərv] | nerve | nervo'muscular |
| sthen- | [sthēn] | strength | 'myasthenia |

*Terminations*

| | | | |
|---|---|---|---|
| -tribe, -trite (trib/e) | [trīb, trīt] | instrument for crushing | 'angiotribe |
| -tripsy (trips/y) | [tripsē] | surgical crushing | 'neurotripsy |
| -mere, -mer (mer/e) | [mər] | part | 'blastomere |

The term cerebellum again illustrates the use of diminutives in medical terminology. Literally the cerebellum is a small brain (from cerebrum), but is used to identify the hind brain. Both the brain and spinal cord are protected by three layers of membrane, the meninges. The outer layer is the dura mater, a Latin phrase meaning hard mother; the middle layer is the arachnoid, named from its web-like appearance (*arachne* is the Greek word for spider); the inner layer is the pia mater, Latin for tender mother.

*Exercise*

Complete the terms below by using the definitions at the right.

1. (dolicho)cephalic — pertaining to a long head
2. (amphibi)ous — pertaining to both (types of) life
3. pre(ganglion)ic — pertaining to (a position) before a ganglion

4. (intraven)ous — within a vein
5. (neur )a(sthenia) — no nerve strength
6. an(encephal )ia — a condition of having no brain
7. litho(tripsy ) — surgical crushing of stones
8. (extra )cystic — outside a bladder
9. electro(encephalograph — a recording of the electrical impulses of the brain
10. (macro )scelia — a condition of large legs

Provide definitions for the following terms.

1. anachronism condition of time again
2. macrophage ______
3. decerebrate ______
4. meningocele ______
5. microcephalic ______
6. myelasthenia ______
7. astrocyte ______
8. encephalosclerosis ______
9. desquamate ______
10. metapyretic ______

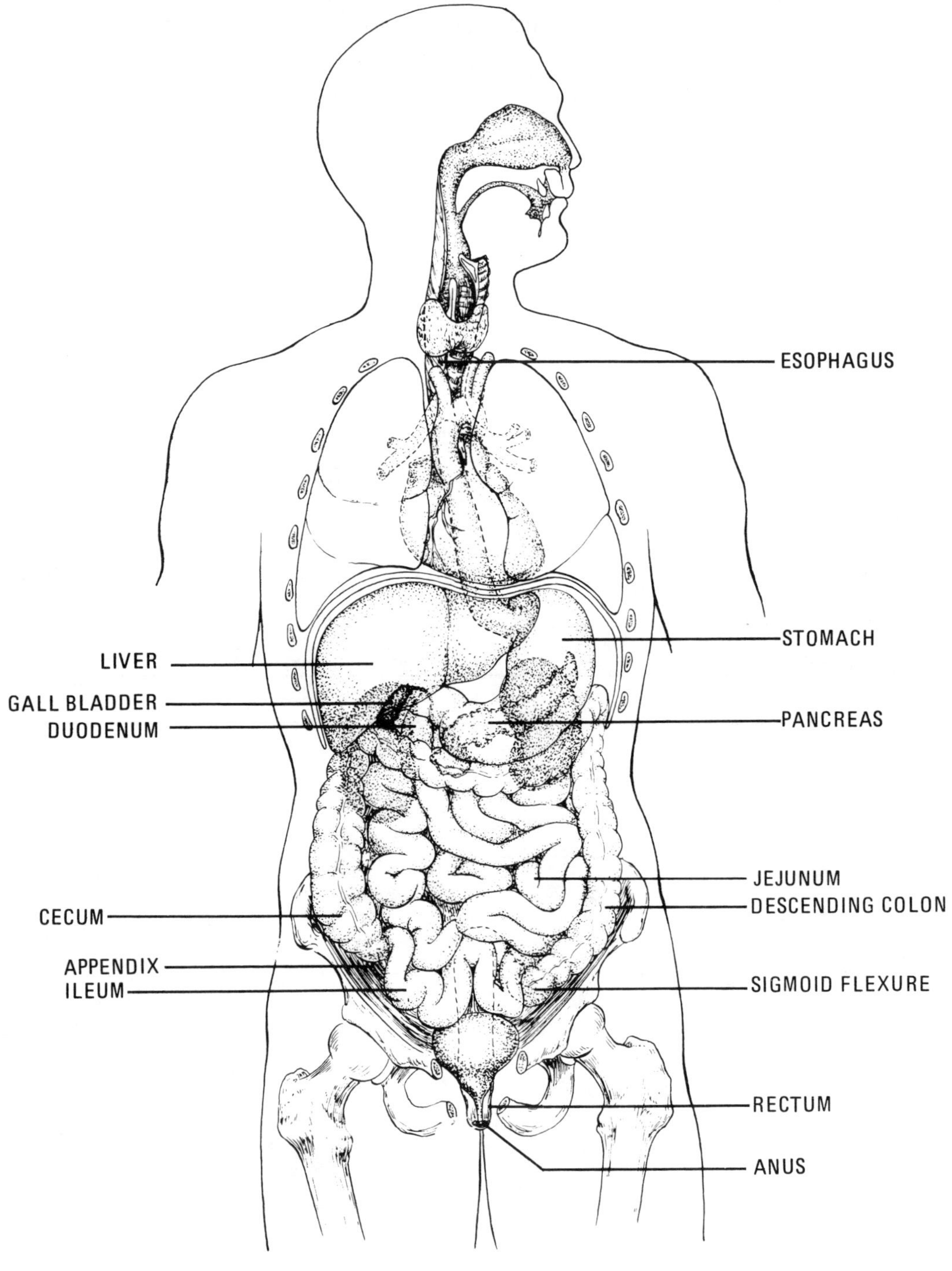
ESOPHAGUS
STOMACH
LIVER
GALL BLADDER
DUODENUM
PANCREAS
JEJUNUM
DESCENDING COLON
CECUM
APPENDIX
ILEUM
SIGMOID FLEXURE
RECTUM
ANUS

PLATE II

# Chapter 6

# DIGESTIVE SYSTEM

| Elements | Pronunciations | Meanings | Examples |
|---|---|---|---|
| *Base Forms* | | | |
| stomat-, stom- | [stōmət] | mouth | stomato'rrhagia |
| *or- | [or] | mouth | oro'nasal |
| cheil- | [kīl] | lip | chei'litis |
| *labi- | [lābē] | lip | labiomy'cosis |
| gloss- | [gläs] | tongue | 'glossocele |
| *lingu- | [lēŋ·gw] | tongue | 'lingual |
| esophag- | [esäfəj] | esophagus | esopha'gismus |
| gastr- | [gas·tr] | stomach | gastrade'nitis |
| pylor- | [pīlor] | pylorus | py'lorospasm |
| hepat- | [hepət] | liver | hepa'tauxe |
| pancreat- | [pankrēat] | pancreas | pancreathel'cosis |
| chol(e)-, chol- | [kol] | bile | cho'lemia |
| cholecyst- | [kolēsist] | gallbladder | cholecystec'tasia |
| choledoch- | [kolēdok] | (common) bile duct | choledocholi'thiasis |
| enter- | [entər] | small intestine | enterel'cosis |
| duoden- | [duədən] | duodenum | duode'noscopy |
| jejun- | [jijūn] | jejunum | jejunoile'ostomy |
| ile- | [ilē] | ileum | ileo'cecal |
| append-, appendic- | [apend] | appendix | appen'dectomy |
| col-, colon- | [kōl] | colon, large intestine | coloente'ritis |
| cec- | [sēk] | cecum | cecop'tosis |
| typhl- | [ti·fl] | cecum | typhloste'nosis |
| sigmoid- | [sigmoyd] | sigmoid flexure | sigmoid'oscopy |
| rect- | [rekt] | rectum | 'rectocele |
| proct- | [präkt] | anus and rectum | proc'toscopy |

| Elements | Pronunciations | Meanings | Examples |
|---|---|---|---|
| an- | [ān] | anus | ano'spinal |
| abdomin- | [abdomin] | abdomen | abdominocen'tesis |
| celi- | [sēlē] | abdominal cavity | celi'orrhaphy |
| lapar- | [lapər] | abdominal wall | laparoneph'rectomy |
| peritone-, periton- | [peritōnē] | peritoneum | peritoneo'clysis |
| oment- | [ōment] | omentum | o'mentopexy |
| epipl- | [epi·pl] | omentum | e'piplocele |
| splanchn- | [splaŋk·n] | internal organs | splanchnop'tosis |
| *viscer- | [visər] | internal organs | viscero'trophic |
| bromat- | [brōmət] | food | broma'tology |
| copr- | [ko·pr] | excrement | copro'philic |
| fec-, fecal- | [fēkəl] | excrement | fecal'uria |
| dips- | [d[illegible]s] | thirst | dipso'therapy |
| cyst- | [sist] | bladder, sac | cholecys'titis |
| doch- | [dok] | duct | choledoch'orrhaphy |

*Terminations*

| | | | |
|---|---|---|---|
| -chezia (chez/ia) | [kēzēə] | defecation | hemato'chezia |
| -emesis (eme/sis) | [eməsis] | vomiting | hyper'emesis |
| -emphraxis (em/phrax/is) | [emfraksis] | obstruction | pancreatem'phraxis |
| -iasis (ia/sis) | [īəsis] | presence of, infestation | nephroli'thiasis |
| -pepsia (peps/ia) | [pepsēə] | digestion | eu'pepsia |
| -stalsis, -stole (stal/sis) | [stälsis, stolē] | contraction | peri'stalsis |
| -stomy (stom/y) | [stəmē] | creation of a (new) opening | co'lostomy |

The termination *-stomy* is derived from the Greek word for mouth, *stoma, stomatos.* In its extended use this termination indicates that a new opening or communication has been established

1. between an internal organ and the exterior of the body (colostomy 'the creation of a new opening between the large intestine and the exterior');

2. between one internal organ and another internal organ (gastroenterostomy 'the creation of a new opening between the stomach and the small intestine');
3. between one section of an organ and another section of the same organ (enteroenterostomy 'the creation of a new opening between one part of the small intestine and another part of the small intestine').

The stomach takes its name from the Greek word for mouth, *stoma.* A more specialized Greek term, *stomachos,* was used to describe the throat and the mouth of an organ such as the stomach. Eventually the term *stomachos* became descriptive of the stomach itself. The pylorus, the lower opening of the stomach, is named from the Greek word for gatekeeper. The duodenum derives its name from its length of approximately twelve (Latin *duodeni*) fingers. The second portion of the small intestine, the jejunum, is named from the Latin word for empty. The first section of the large intestine is named because of its terminating in a closed area. Both in Greek (*typhlon*) and in Latin (*cecum*) it is called blind. The es-like section of the descending colon is named from its resemblance to the Greek letter sigma, and the last section of the large intestine receives its name from its straight (Latin *rectum*) alignment. One of the organs secreting digestive juice is the pancreas. Its name is Greek for all (*pan*) flesh (*creas*).

*Exercise*

Complete the terms below by using the definitions at the right.

| | |
|---|---|
| 1. hemi( ) | excision of half the stomach |
| 2. ( )my( ) | muscle pain in the abdominal cavity (area) |
| 3. hemat( ) | vomiting of blood |
| 4. ( )eurynter | dilator of the anus and rectum |
| 5. ( )clysis | irrigation of the gallbladder |
| 6. ( )a( )ia | no (muscle) tension in the cecum |
| 7. aden( ) | obstruction of a gland |
| 8. amylo( ) | poor starch digestion |
| 9. copr( ) | the presence of excrement in the blood |
| 0. ( )scopy | examination (through) the abdominal wall |

Provide definitions for the following terms.

1. cholangitis ______
2. gastroenteritis ______
3. esophagostenosis ______
4. abdominocentesis ______
5. pancreatemphraxis ______
6. rectostenosis ______

7. microstomous ______________________________

8. cecopexy ______________________________

9. hepatitis ______________________________

10. jejunostomy ______________________________

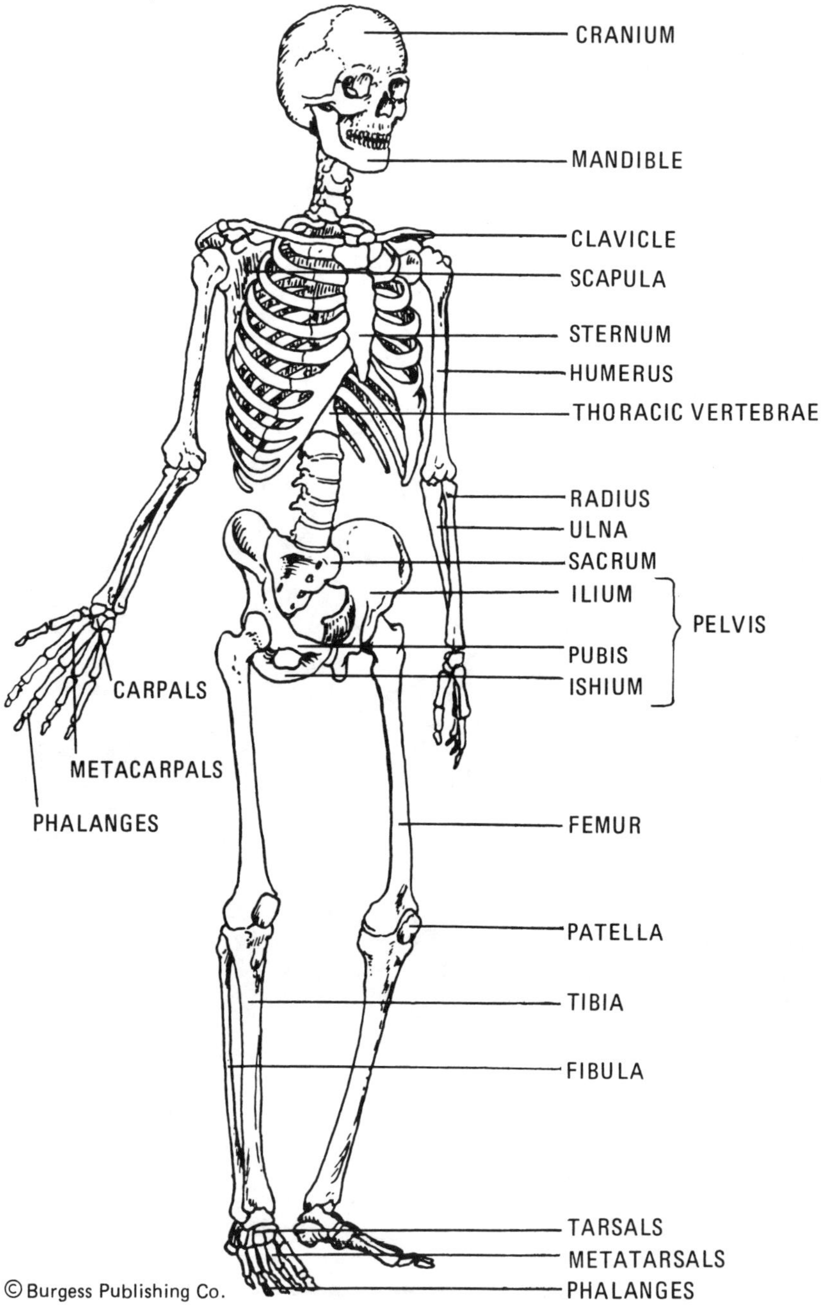
CRANIUM
MANDIBLE
CLAVICLE
SCAPULA
STERNUM
HUMERUS
THORACIC VERTEBRAE
RADIUS
ULNA
SACRUM
ILIUM
PELVIS
PUBIS
ISHIUM
CARPALS
METACARPALS
PHALANGES
FEMUR
PATELLA
TIBIA
FIBULA
TARSALS
METATARSALS
PHALANGES
© Burgess Publishing Co.

PLATE III

# Chapter 7

# SKELETAL SYSTEM

| Elements | Pronunciations | Meanings | Examples |
|---|---|---|---|
| *Prefix* | | | |
| syn-, sym-, syl- | [sin] | with, together | 'symphysis |
| *Base Forms* | | | |
| crani- | [krānē] | skull | crani'ometry |
| clavicul- | [klavikyūl] | clavicle | costocla'vicular |
| scapul- | [skapyul] | scapula | 'scapulopexy |
| acromi- | [akrōmē] | acromium | acromio'humeral |
| humer- | [hyūmər] | humerus | humero'radial |
| radi- | [rādē] | radius | radio'humeral |
| uln- | [uln] | ulna | 'ulnad |
| carp- | [kärp] | carpus | carpometa'carpal |
| phalang- | [fəlanj] | phalanges | hyperpha'langism |
| mandibul- | [mandibyūl] | mandible | man'dibular |
| maxill- | [maksil] | maxilla | maxillo'facial |
| spondyl- | [spändil] | vertebra(e) | spondy'loschisis |
| *vertebr- | [vərtə·br] | vertebra(e) | vertebro'costal |
| stern- | [stərn] | sternum | sternoperi'cardial |
| cost- | [käst] | rib | 'costotome |
| sacr- | [sā·kr] | sacrum | sacrocox'algia |
| coccyg- | [koksij] | coccyx | coccy'gectomy |
| pelv(i)-, pelv- | [pelv] | pelvis | pelviperito'nitis |
| ili- | [ilē] | ilium | ilio'lumbar |
| ischi- | [iskē] | ischium | ischioneu'ralgia |
| pub-, pubi- | [pyūb] | pubis | sub'pubic |

| Elements | Pronunciations | Meanings | Examples |
|---|---|---|---|
| cox- | [koks] | hip joint | cox'itis |
| femor- | [femər] | femur | femoro'tibial |
| patell- | [pətel] | patella | pa'telliform |
| tibi- | [tibē] | tibia | tibio'femoral |
| fibul- | [fibyūl] | fibula | fibulocal'caneal |
| tars- | [tärs] | tarsus | tarsometa'tarsal |
| *astragal- | [astragəl] | astragalus | as'tragalar |
| tal- | [tāl] | talus | talocal'caneal |
| calcane- | [kalkānē] | calcaneum, calcaneus | cal'caneal |
| oste- | [ästē] | bone | osteo'genic |
| myel- | [mīəl] | bone marrow | myelopoi'esis |
| arthr- | [ärth·r] | joint | arth'rotomy |
| articul- | [ärtikyūl] | joint | ar'ticulate |
| burs- | [bərs] | bursa | 'bursolith |
| synovi- | [sinōvē] | synovial fluid, synovial membrane | synovi'oma |
| chondr- | [kän·dr] | cartilage | chon'dropathy |
| condyl- | [kändil] | condyle | 'condyloid |
| tend-, tendin- | [tend] | tendon | ten'dolysis |
| ten-, tenont- | [tenont] | tendon | tenon'titis |
| desm- | [dez·m] | ligament | desmec'tasia |
| rachi-, rach(i)- | [rākē] | spine | rachio'campsia |
| spin- | [spīn] | spine | spi'nalgia |
| fibr- | [fī·br] | fiber | fibrochon'dritis |
| sarc- | [särk] | flesh | sar'cophagy |
| scoli- | [skōlē] | curved, bent | scoli'ometer |

*Suffix*

| | | | |
|---|---|---|---|
| -ar | [ər] | pertaining to | pa'tellar |

| Elements | Pronunciations | Meanings | Examples |
|---|---|---|---|
| *Terminations* | | | |
| -phyte<br>(phy/te) | [fīt] | growth | 'arthrophyte |
| -physis<br>(phy/sis) | [fisis, fīsis] | growing | e'piphysis |
| -thesis<br>(the/sis) | [thēsis] | putting, placing | pros'thesis |
| -osteosis, -ostosis<br>(oste/o/sis) | [ästōsis] | ossification, calcification | sarco'stosis |
| -campsia<br>(camps/ia) | [kampsēə] | bending, curvature | rachio'campsia |
| -clasis, -clasia<br>(cla/sis) | [klāzēə] | fracture | arthro'clasia |
| -necrosis<br>(necr/o/sis) | [nekrōsis] | death, dead condition | cardione'crosis |
| -edema<br>(ede/ma) | [ədēmə] | swelling | acroe'dema |

Many of the terms for bones reflect their resemblance to "household" items. Bursa originally meant a small bag, clavicle (a diminutive of the Latin *clavis*) a small key, fibula a brooch, patella a shallow dish, pelvis a basin, and tibia a flute. The phalanges bear the Greek name for the close ordered ranks of a battle line, a phalanx.

The term hypochondria reflects an old belief that moods or humors were resident in an area of the body below the cartilage of the breastbone. While the term originally referred to gloominess or melancholy it has today come to mean an exaggerated anxiety about one's health.

*Exercise*

Complete the terms below by using the definitions at the right.

| | | |
|---|---|---|
| 1. | ( )arthr( ) | inflammation of joint bones |
| 2. | ( )syndesis | binding together of vertebrae |
| 3. | ( )dys( ) | poor ossification of the skull |
| 4. | syn( )physis | growing together of joints |
| 5. | ( )lith | calculus in a bursa |
| 6. | ( )ar | pertaining to the patella |
| 7. | arthr( ) | swelling of a joint |
| 8. | ( )oid | resembling cartilage |
| 9. | ( )sarcoma | a flesh tumor of the bone |
| 10. | ( )optosis | prolapse of the tarsal bones |

Provide definitions for the following terms.

1. exostosis ____________________
2. chrondromalacia ____________________
3. osteoclasis ____________________
4. arthroplasty ____________________
5. osteogenic ____________________
6. osteonecrosis ____________________
7. desmorrhexis ____________________
8. myeloblast ____________________
9. interphalangeal ____________________
10. pelvimetry ____________________

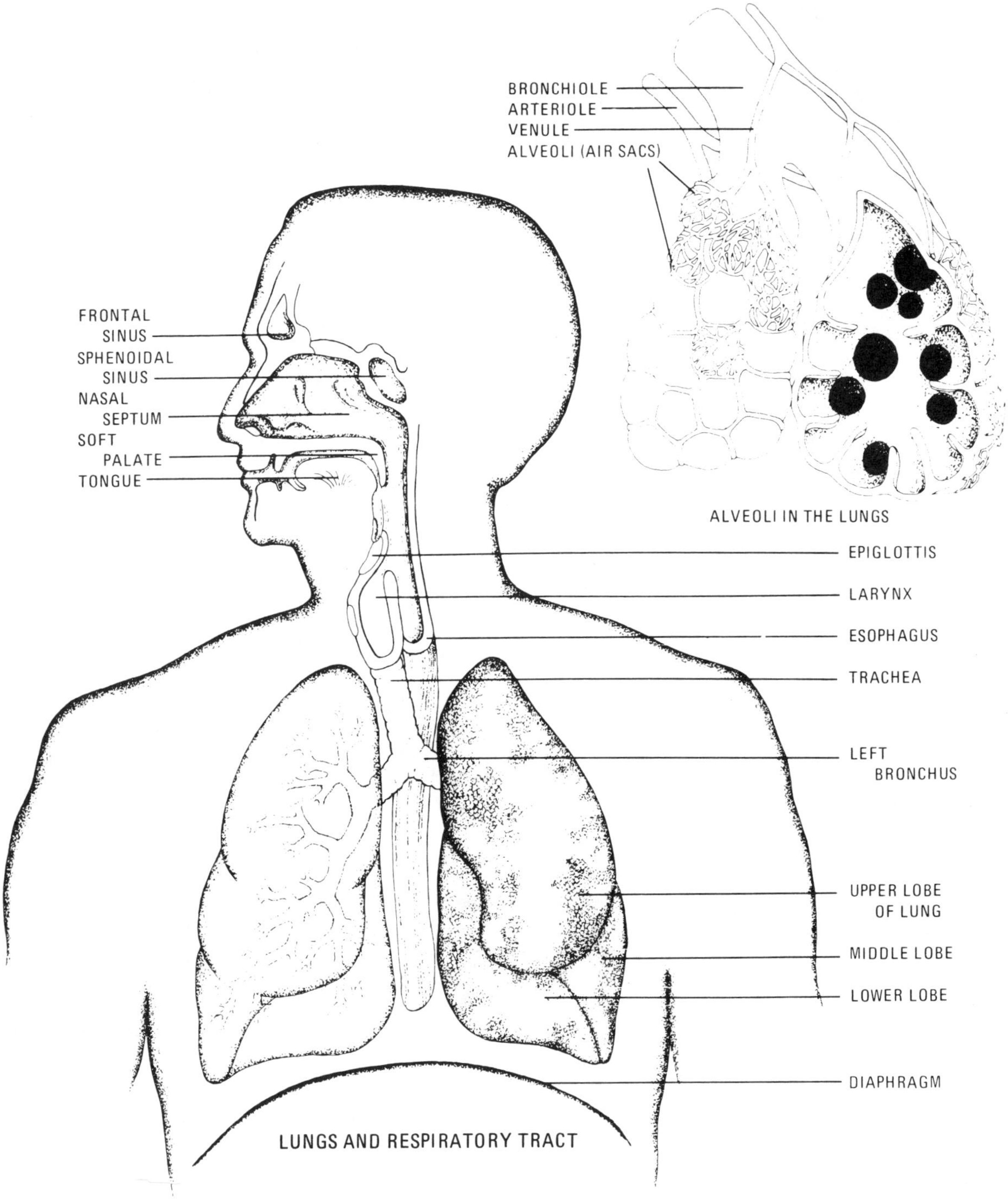


LUNGS AND RESPIRATORY TRACT



**PLATE IV**

# Chapter 8 (31)

# RESPIRATORY SYSTEM

| Elements | Pronunciations | Meanings | Examples |
|---|---|---|---|
| *Prefix* | | | |
| epi- | [epē, epə] | upon, over | epi'dermic |
| *Base Forms* | | | |
| rhin- | [rīn] | nose | rhino'megaly |
| nas-, nas(i)- | [nāz] | nose | 'nasoscope |
| nar(i)- | [nar] | nostril | 'narial |
| sept-, sept(i)- | [sept] | septum | nasosep'titis |
| sin-, sinus- | [sīn] | sinus | 'sinogram |
| antr- | [an·tr] | cavity | nasoan'tritis |
| pharyng- | [farin·g] | pharynx | pharyngo'keratosis |
| epiglott-, epiglottid- | [epēglät] | epiglottis | epiglotti'ditis |
| glott- | [glät] | glottis | 'glottic |
| laryng- | [larin·g] | larynx | la'ryngospasm |
| chord- | [kord] | (vocal) cord | chor'ditis |
| trache- | [trākē] | trachea | tracheopy'osis |
| bronch-, bronchi- | [bräŋkē] | bronchus | bronchi'ectasis |
| bronchiol- | [bräŋkēol] | bronchiole | bronchio'litis |
| pneum- | [nūm] | air, lung | pneumody'namics |
| pneumon- | [nūmōn] | lung | pneumon'emia |
| pulm-, pulmon- | [pulmōn] | lung | pulmo'nitis |
| pleur- | [plūr] | pleura | pleurocen'tesis |
| phren- | [fren] | diaphragm | phrenocolo'pexy |
| pne- | [nē] | breathe | pne'ometer |
| aer- | [āer, er] | air | 'aerocele |

| Elements | Pronunciations | Meanings | Examples |
|---|---|---|---|
| pneumat- | [nūmat] | air, gas | pneu'matocele |
| coni- | [kōnē] | dust | pneumoconi'osis |
| xer- | [zir] | dry | xeroph'thalmia |
| tuss- | [təs] | cough | 'tussal |
| thorac- | [thōrak] | thorax | thora'cometry |
| *Suffix* | | | |
| -ism | [izum] | state, condition | poly'dactylism |
| *Terminations* | | | |
| -ismus (ism/us) | [izmus] | spasm | laryn'gismus |
| -rrhagia (rrhag/ia) | [rājēə] | hemorrhage | rhino'rrhagia |
| -pnea (pne/a) | [p·nēə] | breathing | hyper'phea |

The diaphragm (Greek *dia* across and *phragma* fence) separates the abdomen from the thoracic cavity. The Greek word *thorax* described the breastplate worn by Greek warriors and the area of the chest protected by it. The term septum is borrowed from the Latin word meaning wall, fence, or enclosure.

*Exercise*

Complete the terms below by using the definitions at the right.

| | Term | Definition |
|---|---|---|
| 1. | ( xero )cheilia | condition of dry lips |
| 2. | (antituss)ive | (acting) against a cough |
| 3. | broncho( rrhagia ) | hemorrhage of the bronchi |
| 4. | (pneumo)lith( iasis ) | presence of calculus in the lungs |
| 5. | ( sinus )itis | inflammation of the sinuses |
| 6. | eu( pnea ) | breathing normally |
| 7. | ( rhino )rrhagia | hemorrhage of the nose |
| 8. | (aerodermo)ectasia | dilatation of the skin by air |

9. (dys)pnea — painful breathing
10. (trache)otomy — incision of the trachea

Provide definitions for the following terms.

1. bronchitis ________________________________
2. pneumonectomy ________________________________
3. epidermic ________________________________
4. nasopharyngitis ________________________________
5. laryngectomy ________________________________
6. pneumoconiosis ________________________________
7. nasogastric ________________________________
8. pharyngismus ________________________________
9. endotracheal ________________________________
10. atelectasis ________________________________

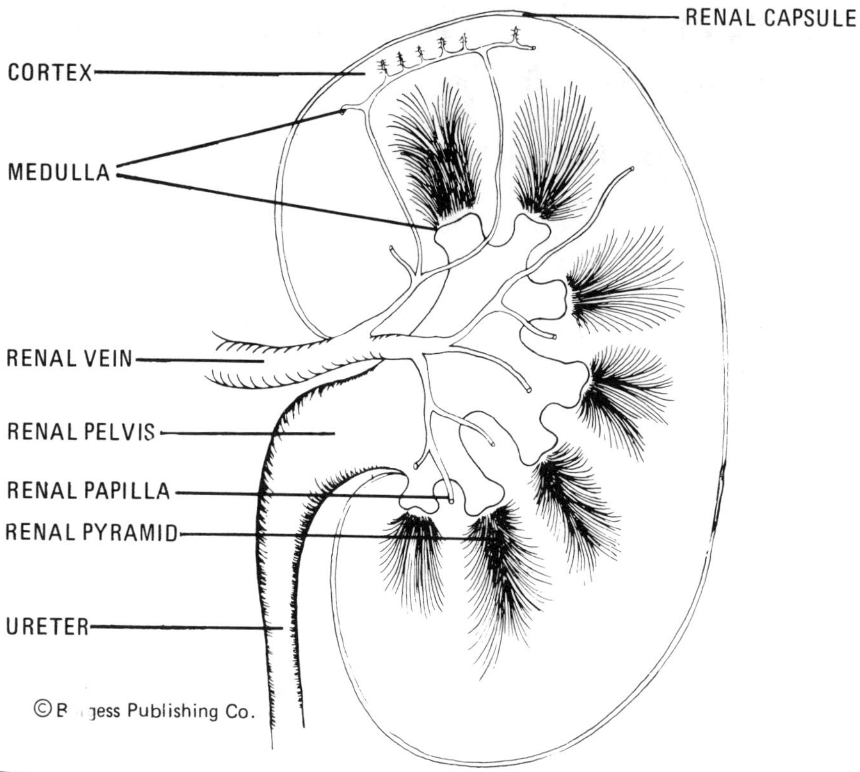
RENAL CAPSULE
CORTEX
MEDULLA
RENAL VEIN
RENAL PELVIS
RENAL PAPILLA
RENAL PYRAMID
URETER
©B  gess Publishing Co.

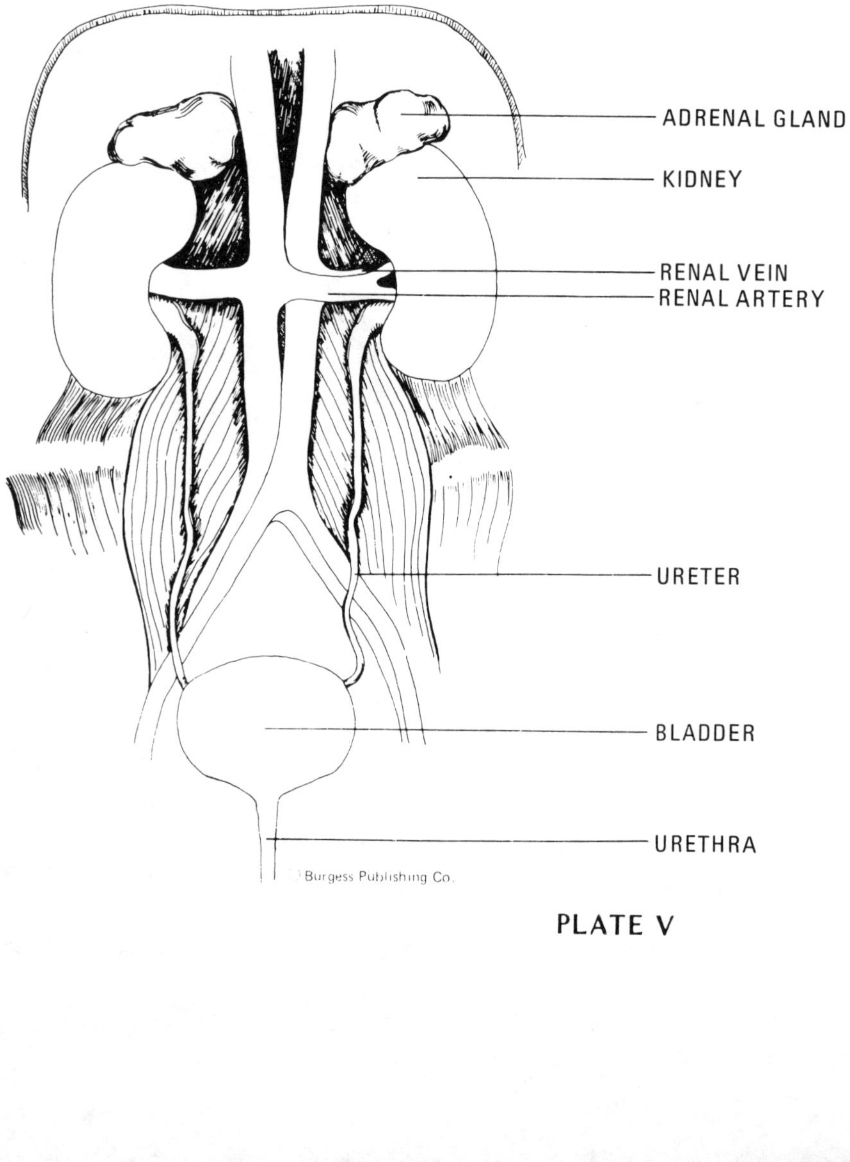
ADRENAL GLAND
KIDNEY
RENAL VEIN
RENAL ARTERY
URETER
BLADDER
URETHRA
Burgess Publishing Co.

PLATE V

## Chapter 9 (25)

# URINARY SYSTEM

| Elements | Pronunciations | Meanings | Examples |
|---|---|---|---|
| *Prefixes* | | | |
| juxta- | [jəkstə] | close to | juxtaglo'merular |
| apo- | [apō] | from, away | aponeu'rosis |
| con-, com-, col- | [kän] | with, together, completely | consan'guineous |
| contra-, contro- | [käntrə] | opposite, against | contra'lateral |
| retro- | [retrō] | backward | retro'plasia |
| ultra- | [ultrə] | beyond | ultrabrachyce'phalic |
| ambi- | [ambē] | both | ambi'dextrous |
| eu- | [yū] | good, well | eu'pepsia |
| per- | [per] | through, completely | per'oral |
| *Base Forms* | | | |
| glomerul- | [glomeryul] | glomerulus | glomerulone'phritis |
| nephr- | [ne·fr] | kidney | nephroscler'osis |
| ren-, ren(i)- | [rēn] | kidney | re'nopathy |
| pyel- | [pīel] | renal pelvis | pyelolith'otomy |
| ureter- | [yūrētər] | ureter | uretero'rrhagia |
| cyst- | [sist] | bladder, sac | 'cystoscope |
| *vesic- | [vesik] | bladder, sac | vesi'cotomy |
| urethr- | [yūrēth·r] | urethra | urethro'staxis |
| meat- | [mēət] | meatus, opening | mea'toscopy |
| ur- | [yur] | urine | urocyan'osis |
| olig- | [olēg] | little, few | oligohy'druria |
| pol(y)- | [polē] | much, many | polyhy'druria |

| Elements | Pronunciations | Meanings | Examples |
|---|---|---|---|
| *Terminations* | | | |
| -eurynter (euryn/ter) | [yurintər] | dilator | col'peurynter |
| -staxis (stax/is) | [staksis] | dripping, oozing | cysto'staxis |
| -schesis, -schesia (sche/sis) | [skesis] | suppression, retention | u'roschesis |
| -uria (ur/ia) | [yurēə] | urine condition | lith'uria |

*Exercise*

Complete the terms below by using the definitions at the right.

1. hemat( uria ) — the presence of blood in urine
2. aero(urethro)scopy — examination of the urethra (using) air
3. uro(cyanosis) — abnormal condition of blue urine
4. urethr(emphraxis) — obstruction of the urethra
5. (nephro )hyper( trophy ) — excessive development of the kidneys
6. (pyelo )gram — a recording of the renal pelvis
7. py(uria ) — the presence of pus in urine
8. ( poly )uria — a condition of much urine
9. (cyst )oid — bladder-like
10. uro(poiesis ) — urine production

Provide definitions for the following terms.

1. apophysis ____________________
2. ureterolith ____________________
3. cyanuria ____________________
4. cystolithiasis ____________________
5. uropenia ____________________
6. nephroptosis ____________________
7. dysuria ____________________
8. transurethral ____________________
9. oligopepsia ____________________
10. cystitis ____________________

# REVIEW A

Review A consists of fifty terms which reflect the elements introduced in the first nine chapters. Write the definitions for these terms in the spaces provided and then check your answers by consulting the indices in the back of the text.

angiasthenia condition of weak vessels

anisopiesis condition of unequal pressure

antilithic preventing the formation of stones

atelomyelia condition of incomplete spinal chord develop.

cardioptosis sagging heart

cephalocentesis surgical punture of the head

cholelithotripsy surgical crushing of gall (bile) stones

chromaturia condition of abnormally colored urine

dyskinesia loss of ability to do poor movement

dysphemia poor speech (disorder)

encephalatrophy wasting away of the brain

epigastralgia pain over the stomach (hindgut)

erythrocyanosis abnormal condition of bluish-red [color of skin]

hematostatic pertaining to stopping (stagnation) of blood

hepatogenous caused by [produced in] the liver

hydrophilous pertaining to love of water [water absorbing]

hyperlipemia blood condition of excessive [fat]

hyperpnea excessive breathing rate

hypnophobia condition of fearing sleep

hypodermatoclysis [replace] deficient water after illness washing out of below the skin

ileostomy creation of a new hole in the ileum

interchondral pertaining to between cartiledges

laryngitis inflammation of the larynx

leukocytopoiesis ______ production of w.b.c.

lipolysis ______ destruction ~~degradation~~ or dissolution ~~destruction~~ of fats

lithonephrotomy ______ removal of kidney stones
incision, dividing stone

lymphagogue ______ agent inducing flow [production]] of lymph

microglossia ______ condition of small tongue

myocardial ______ pertaining to heart muscles

myxorrhea ______ a flow of mucus

nasoseptitis ______ inflammation of nasal septum

neostomy ______ [surgical] creation of a new opening

nephremphraxis ______ obstruction of the kidneys

nephrotoxin ______ poison of the kidney (effects kidney)

osteoarthropathy ______ a disease of the bone + joints

panneuritis ______ inflammation of (multiple) all nerves

parachromatosis ______ abnormal condition of abnormal color

paracolitis ______ inflammation of outer coat of colon

photodynamic ______ pertaining to power of light

pneumogalactocele [tumor w/ gas + milk]
swelling w/ " " "

polyphobia fear of many things

proctopexy fixation of anus + rectum
[" " " to adj. organ or tissue]

pyochezia defecation of pus
[pus in stool]

rachitome instrument to cut the spine

splanchnosclerosis hardening of the internal organs

splenectasia dilatation/stretching of the spleen

spondyloschisis splitting of the vertebrae

tachyphagia condition of rapid eating

thrombectomy surgical excision of a clot

urologist one who specializes in the study of urine, (tract, etc.)

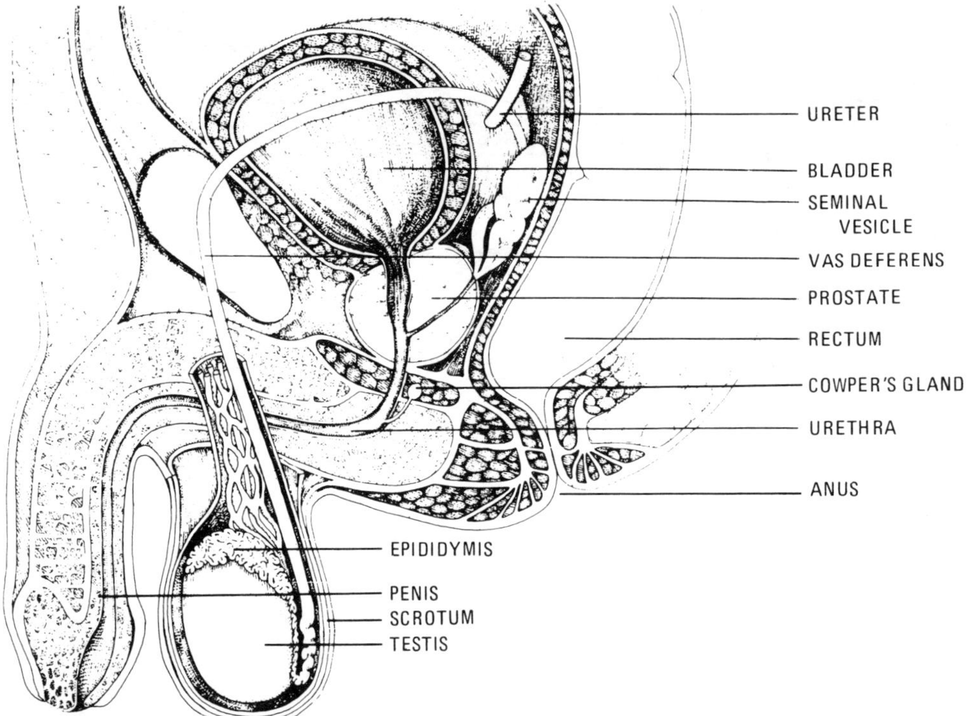




HUMAN MALE REPRODUCTIVE SYSTEM

**PLATE VI**

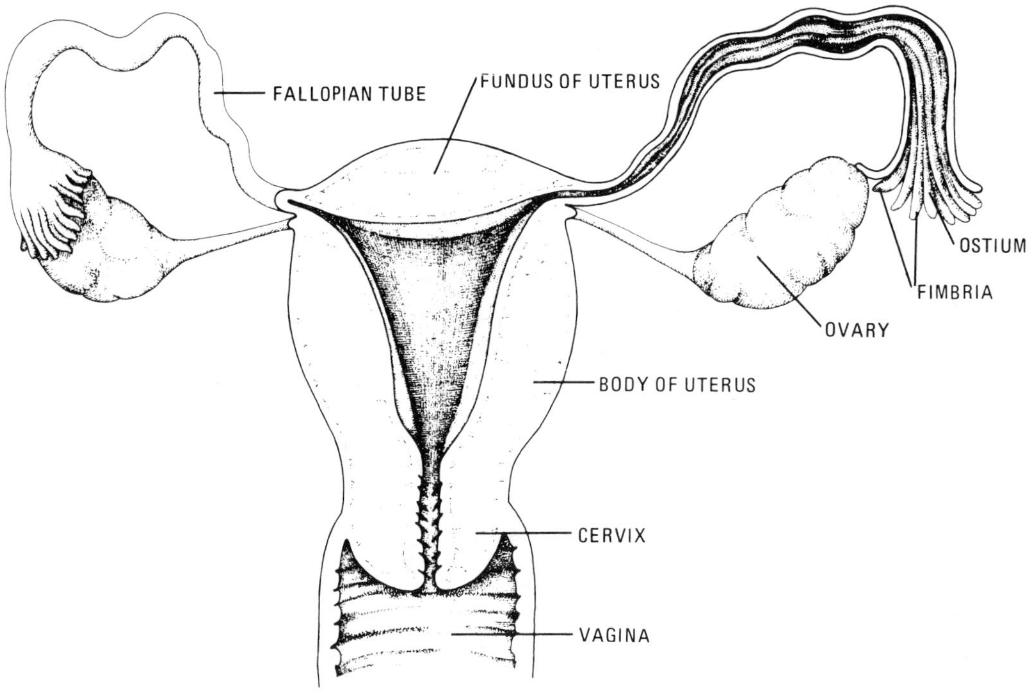




HUMAN FEMALE REPRODUCTIVE SYSTEM

**PLATE VII**

# Chapter 10

# GENITAL SYSTEM

| Elements | Pronunciations | Meanings | Examples |
|---|---|---|---|
| *Male Reproductive System* | | | |
| scrot- | [skrōt] | scrotum | 'scrotocele |
| osche- | [oskē] | scrotum | osche'oncus |
| orchi-, orchid- | [orkid] | testicle | orchidop'tosis |
| test-, test(i)- | [test] | testicle | tes'tectomy |
| epididym- | [epēdidəm] | epididymis | epididy'mitis |
| vas- | [vas] | vas deferens | vaso'section |
| prostat- | [prostat] | prostate gland | prosta'totomy |
| phall- | [fal] | penis | phallo'rrhagia |
| pen-, pen(i)- | [pēn] | penis | pen'ischisis |
| balan- | [balan] | glans penis | ba'lanic |
| sperm-, spermat- | [spərmət] | sperm, seed | sperma'tolysis |
| semin- | [semin] | semen | 'seminal |
| *Female Reproductive System* | | | |
| o- | [ō] | egg, ovum | 'oocyst |
| ov(i)-, ov- | [ōv] | egg, ovum | o'viferous |
| oophor- | [ōofor] | ovary | oopho'roma |
| salping- | [salpiŋ·g] | fallopian tube | salpingocy'esis |
| uter- | [yūtər] | uterus | utero'tonic |
| metr- | [mē·tr] | uterus | metrec'tasia |
| hyster- | [histər] | uterus | hyster'ometry |
| cervic- | [servik] | cervix | cervicovagi'nitis |
| trachel- | [trākel] | cervix | trachel'ectomy |
| colp- | [kolp] | vagina | colpa'tresia |

| Elements | Pronunciations | Meanings | Examples |
|---|---|---|---|
| vagin- | [vajin] | vagina | 'vaginoscope |
| men- | [men] | menses, menstruation | meno'staxis |
| *General Forms* | | | |
| andr- | [an·dr] | man, male | 'android |
| gyn-, gynec- | [gīnək] | woman, female | gyne'cologist |
| gam- | [gam] | marriage | mo'nogamy |
| fet- | [fēt] | fetus | fe'tometry |
| amni- | [amnē] | amnion, amniotic fluid | amnio'rrhexis |
| par- | [par] | give birth | paro'dynia |
| toc- | [tōs, tōk] | childbirth | dys'tocia |
| carcin- | [kärsin] | cancer | carcino'genic |
| crypt- | [kript] | hidden | cryptomeno'rrhea |
| *Terminations* | | | |
| -gravida (gravid/a) | [gravidə] | a woman who is pregnant | multi'gravida |
| -para (par/a) | [pərə] | a woman who has given birth | nul'lipara |
| -cyesis (cye/sis) | [sīēsis] | pregnancy | pseudocy'esis |

The epididymis is named from its location upon the testes, the Greek word *didymos* meaning twin and then testicle. Testicle, a diminutive of the Latin *testis,* witness, has come to be applied to the male sex glands since they give evidence of manhood. The element men- is derived from the Greek words for month and moon, while the terms menses and menstruation are taken from the Latin *mensis,* month. The monthly occurrence of the menstrual cycle thus led to its terminology. The fallopian tubes are named from their resemblance to the Greek war trumpet, *salpinx.* Hysteria, a uterine condition according to the meaning of its elements, was so named because behavior of an excited sort was thought to reflect disorders of the female reproductive system.

*Exercise*

Provide medical terms which correspond to the following definitions.

1. a scrotal tumor ______
2. flow from the penis ______
3. the presence of sperm in urine ______
4. excision of (a section of) the vas deferens ______
5. a vaginal dilator ______
6. painful menstrual flow ______
7. fixation of an ovary ______
8. the condition of hidden testicles ______
9. marriage outside (the tribe) ______
10. giving birth through eggs ______
11. a condition of hidden menses ______
12. pregnancy within a fallopian tube ______
13. surgical puncture (to withdraw) amniotic fluid ______
14. hemorrhage of the uterus ______
15. a condition of no sperm ______
16. a condition of no testicles ______
17. little menstrual flow ______
18. slow childbirth ______
19. suppression of sperm ______
20. semen bearing ______

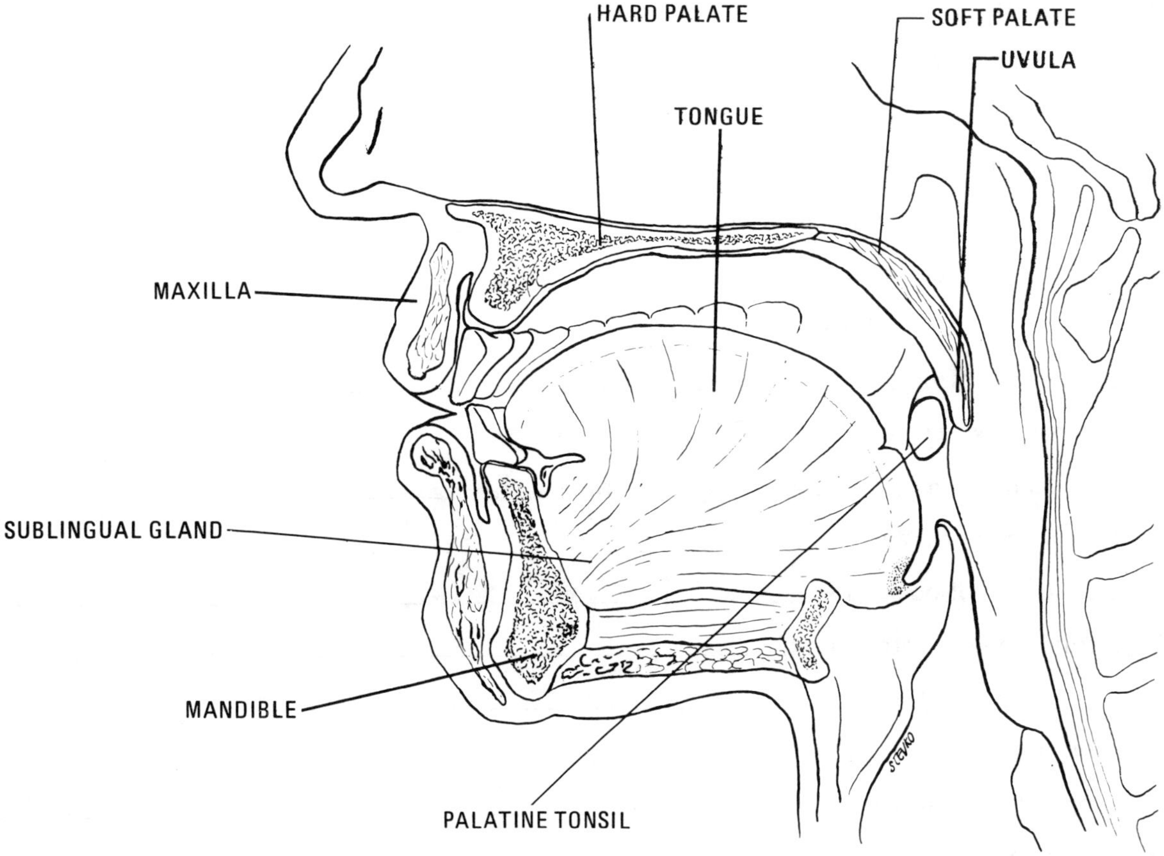
HARD PALATE
SOFT PALATE
UVULA
TONGUE
MAXILLA
SUBLINGUAL GLAND
MANDIBLE
PALATINE TONSIL
STEVKO

**PLATE VIII**

# Chapter 11

# ORAL-DENTAL FORMS

| Elements | Pronunciations | Meanings | Examples |
|---|---|---|---|
| *Prefixes* | | | |
| peri- | [perē] | around | perio'dontal |
| pros- | [präs] | toward, in addition | pros'thesis |
| *Base Forms* | | | |
| cheil- | [kīl] | lip | 'cheiloplasty |
| labi- | [lābē] | lip | labiomy'cosis |
| maxill- | [maksil] | maxilla | maxillo'facial |
| mandibul- | [mandibyūl] | mandible | man'dibular |
| bucc- | [buk] | cheek | 'buccal |
| gnath- | [nath] | jaw | 'gnathoplasty |
| or- | [or] | mouth | oro'lingual |
| stomat-, stom- | [stōmət] | mouth | stoma'topathy |
| odont- | [ōdänt] | tooth | odonto'therapy |
| dent(i)-, dent- | [dent] | tooth | 'dentate |
| adamantin-, adamant- | [adəmant] | enamel | ada'mantoblast |
| amel- | [amel] | enamel | amelo'dentinal |
| dentin- | [dentin] | dentin | dentino'genic |
| cuspid- | [kəspid] | point | tri'cuspid |
| alveol- | [alvēol] | tooth socket | alveo'litis |
| gingiv- | [jinjiv] | gum | gingiv'algia |
| *ul- | [yūl] | gum | u'litis |
| gloss- | [gläs] | tongue | 'glossocele |
| lingu- | [lēŋ·gw] | tongue | 'linguiform |

| Examples | Pronunciations | Meanings | Examples |
|---|---|---|---|
| fren- | [fren] | frenum, frenulum | 'frenal |
| palat- | [palət] | (hard) palate | 'palatal |
| uranisc-, uran- | [yūran] | (hard) palate | uran'oschisis |
| staphyl- | [stafil] | soft palate | 'staphyloplasty |
| vel- | [vēl] | velum | 'velarize |
| uvul-, uvul(a)- | [yūvyəl] | uvula | 'uvulatome |
| orth- | [orth] | straight | ortho'dontist |
| schiz-, schist- | [skist] | split | schisto'glossia |
| apic- | [āpik] | apex, tip | apic'ectomy |

*Termination*

| | | | |
|---|---|---|---|
| -schisis | [skisis] | splitting | cheilognathopala'to-schisis |

Permanent teeth are of four types. The incisors are literally cutters, the molars are grinders, the bicuspids are two pointed. The last type, the canines, are named after their resemblance to dogs' teeth.

The hard palate, the domed roof of the mouth, has taken its name from the Greek for sky, *uranos.* The soft palate has acquired both its Greek and Latin elements from its resemblance in shape to a bunch of grapes, Greek *staphyle,* Latin *uva.* The term velum is the Latin word for veil.

*Exercise*

Provide definitions for the following terms.

1. frenotomy ______
2. gingivitis ______
3. gnathoschisis ______
4. xerocheilia ______
5. labiodental ______
6. odontatrophy ______
7. velosynthesis ______
8. uvuloptosis ______
9. periapical ______
10. odontonecrosis ______

11. uranostaphyloplasty ______
12. perioral ______
13. ulitis ______
14. oronasal ______
15. staphyledema ______
16. ulorrhea ______
17. pedodontist ______
18. sublingual ______
19. postoral ______
20. schistoglossia ______

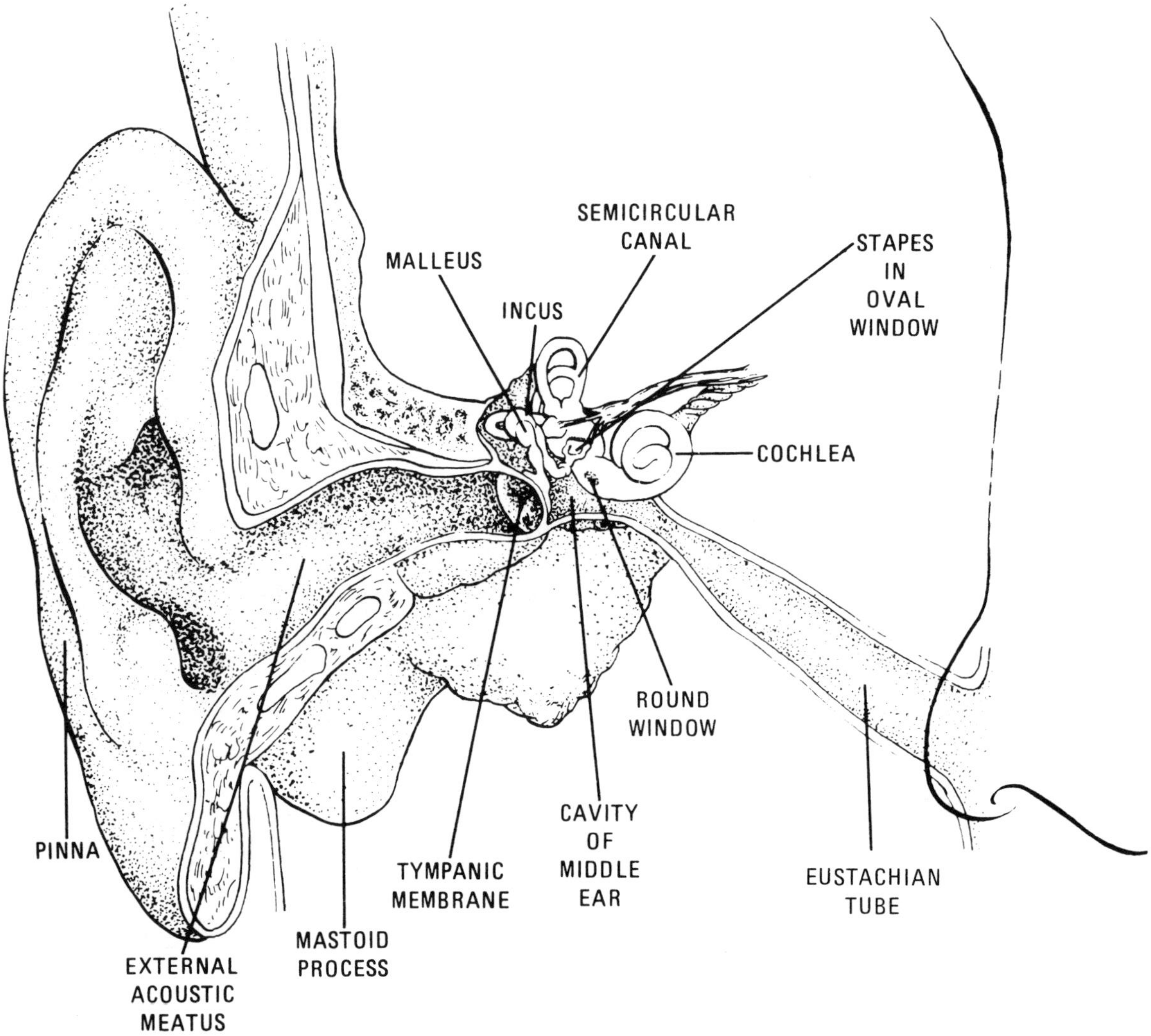
SEMICIRCULAR CANAL
MALLEUS
STAPES IN OVAL WINDOW
INCUS
COCHLEA
ROUND WINDOW
CAVITY OF MIDDLE EAR
PINNA
TYMPANIC MEMBRANE
EUSTACHIAN TUBE
MASTOID PROCESS
EXTERNAL ACOUSTIC MEATUS

**PLATE IX**

# Chapter 12

# EAR-EYE FORMS

| Elements | Pronunciations | Meanings | Examples |
|---|---|---|---|
| *Prefix* | | | |
| eso- | [esō] | inward | eso'tropia |
| | | | |
| *Base Forms* | | | |
| *Ear Forms* | | | |
| ot- | [ōt] | ear | otopyo'rrhea |
| mastoid- | [mastoyd] | mastoid process | mastoidocen'tesis |
| aur(i)-, aur- | [or] | ear | 'auriscope |
| pinn- | [pin] | pinna | 'pinnate |
| meat- | [mēāt] | opening, passage | me'atal |
| myring- | [miriŋ·g] | tympanic membrane | myrin'gotomy |
| tympan- | [timpan] | tympanum | tympan'otomy |
| malle- | [malē] | malleus | malleoin'cudal |
| incud- | [inkūd] | incus | in'cudiform |
| staped- | [stāpēd] | stapes | stape'dectomy |
| eustach- | [yūstāsh] | eustachian tube | eu'stachian |
| labyrinth- | [labərinth] | labyrinth | labyrin'thitis |
| vestibul- | [vestibyūl] | vestibule | vestibulo'cochlear |
| utricul- | [yūtrikyūl] | utricle | utricu'litis |
| fenestr- | [fenə·str] | window | 'fenestrate |
| cochle- | [käklē] | cochlea | 'cochlear |
| acou-, acu- | [əkū] | hear | a'cousia |
| audi-, audit- | [odē] | hear | audi'ology |

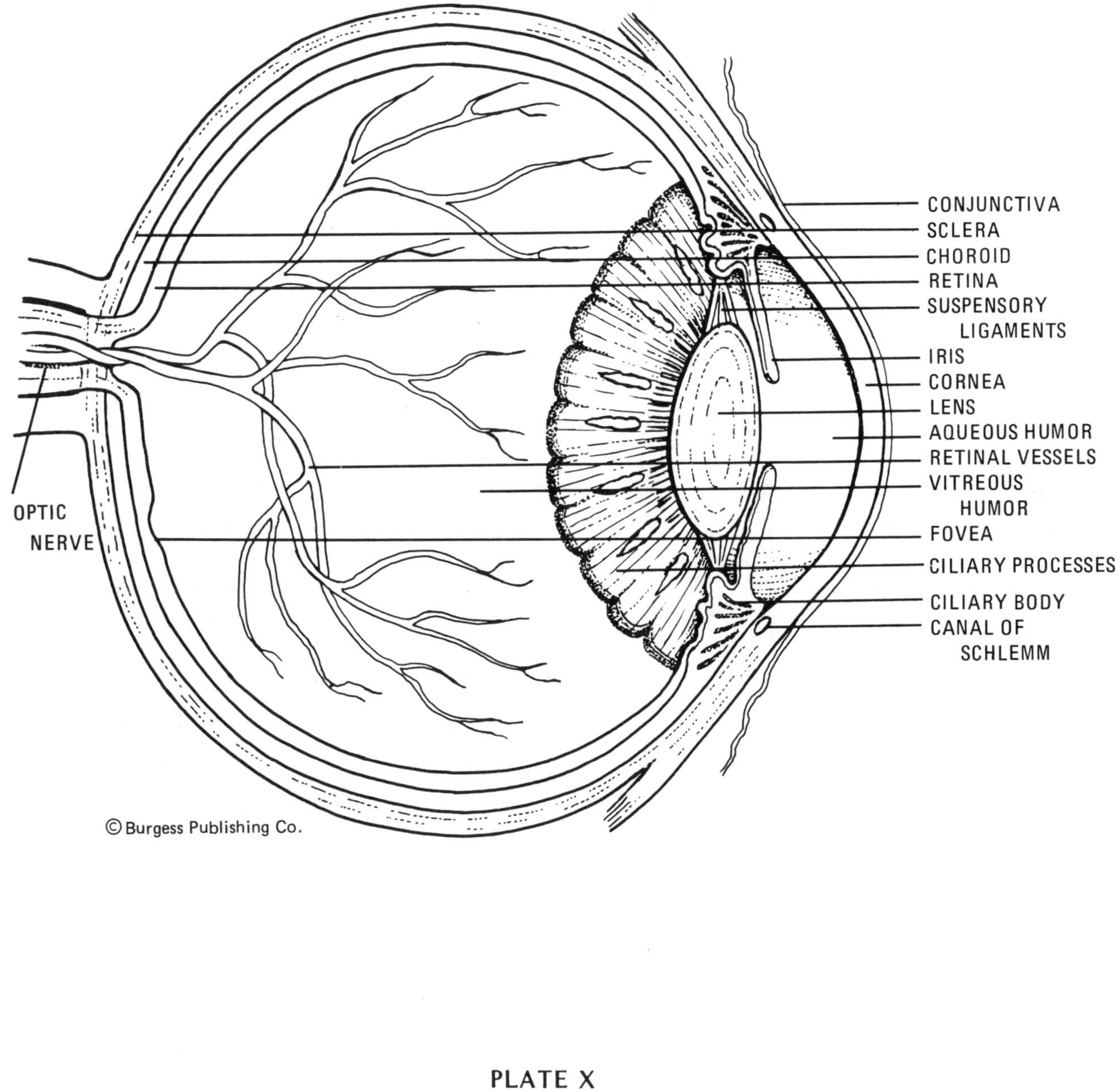
CONJUNCTIVA
SCLERA
CHOROID
RETINA
SUSPENSORY LIGAMENTS
IRIS
CORNEA
LENS
AQUEOUS HUMOR
RETINAL VESSELS
VITREOUS HUMOR
FOVEA
CILIARY PROCESSES
CILIARY BODY
CANAL OF SCHLEMM
OPTIC NERVE



PLATE X

| Elements | Pronunciations | Meanings | Examples |
|---|---|---|---|
| *Eye Forms* | | | |
| ophthalm- | [ofthälm] | eye | oph'thalmia |
| ocul- | [okyūl] | eye | oculo'gyric |
| palpebr- | [palpē·br] | eyelid | 'palpebrate |
| blephar- | [blefər] | eyelid | blepharopa'chynsis |
| cili- | [silē] | eyelash | 'ciliate |
| supercili- | [sūpərsilē] | eyebrow | super'ciliary |
| dacry- | [dakrē] | tear, tear duct | 'dacryolith |
| lacrim- | [lakrim] | tear, tear duct | lacri'mation |
| conjunctiv- | [känjəŋtiv] | conjunctiva | conjunctiv'oma |
| corne- | [kornē] | cornea | corneo'sclera |
| kerat- | [kerət] | cornea | keratohel'cosis |
| ir-, irid- | [irid] | iris | i'ridocele |
| cor-, core- | [korē] | pupil | core'ometry |
| pupill- | [pyūpil] | pupil | pupill'ometer |
| cycl- | [si·kl] | ciliary body | cyclo'plegia |
| lent-, lent(i)- | [lent] | lens | 'lentiform |
| lenticul- | [lentikyūl] | lens | len'ticular |
| phac- | [fak] | lens | phacoglau'coma |
| scler- | [sklēr] | sclera | sclero'cornea |
| uve- | [yūvē] | uveal tract | uve'itis |
| choroid- | [koroyd] | choroid | choroidoretin'itis |
| retin- | [retin] | retina | reti'nopathy |
| stigmat- | [stigmət] | mark, focus point | 'stigmatism |
| gyr- | [jīr] | orbit, circle | ophthalmo'gyric |
| opt- | [äpt] | vision | 'optic |
| blep-, bleps- | [bleps] | vision | para'blepsia |
| ambl(y)- | [amblē] | dull | 'amblyoscope |
| dipl- | [di·pl] | double | diplo'coria |
| *Termination* | | | |
| -opia, opsia (op/ia) | [ōpēə] | vision | dys'opia |

Perhaps the most colorful etymology concerning medical terms involves the element core-. The Greek word *core* means girl or doll. It has become associated with the pupil of the eye because a doll-like image of what is seen appears within the pupil. The word pupil, a diminutive of the Latin word *pupa,* girl or doll, reflects the same etymological process.

Terms relating to parts of the ear are often the names of more familiar objects. Thus the Latin *incus* also means anvil, *malleus* hammer, *stapes* stirrup, *tympanum* drum, and *cochlea* a snail with a spiral shell. The Greek word *labyrinthos* refers to a maze.

*Exercise*

Provide medical terms which correspond to the following definitions.

1. sagging of the eyelid__________
2. dilatation of the pupils__________
3. double vision__________
4. one who specializes in the study of eyes__________
5. incision of the mastoid process__________
6. inflammation of the ear__________
7. deficient hearing__________
8. abnormal condition of eyelids being (joined) together__________
9. displacement of the pupils__________
10. narrowing of the tear ducts__________
11. condition of unequal pupils__________
12. dry eye condition__________
13. flow from the ear__________
14. within the eye__________
15. large ear condition__________
16. no color vision__________
17. hardening (within the) ear__________
18. a condition of no lens__________
19. abnormal condition of fungus on the tympanic membrane__________
20. softening of the lens__________

# Chapter 13

# EXTERNAL ANATOMY

| Elements | Pronunciations | Meanings | Examples |
|---|---|---|---|
| *Base Forms* | | | |
| trich- | [trik] | hair | 'trichoid |
| capit-, -cipit- | [kapit] | head | 'capitate |
| cephal- | [sefəl] | head | cephalohe'mometer |
| faci- | [fāshē] | face | facio'plegia |
| prosop- | [prosōp] | face | prosoponeu'ralgia |
| ment- | [ment] | chin | 'mental |
| cervic- | [servik] | neck | cervico'facial |
| trachel- | [trākel] | neck | trachelo'dynia |
| om- | [ōm] | shoulder | omo'dynia |
| axill- | [aksil] | armpit | 'axillary |
| brachi- | [brākē] | arm | brachio'crural |
| chir-, cheir- | [kīr] | hand | chiro'megaly |
| manu- | [manyū] | hand | bi'manual |
| dactyl- | [daktil] | finger, toe | 'dactylospasm |
| digit- | [dijit] | finger, toe | 'digitate |
| onych- | [onik] | nail | ony'cholysis |
| pector- | [pektər] | chest | pector'algia |
| steth- | [steth] | chest | steth'ometer |
| thorac- | [thōrak] | chest | thoracocen'tesis |
| mamm(i)-, mamm- | [mam] | breast | mam'mography |
| mast-, maz- | [mast] | breast | mast'auxe |
| papill- | [papil] | nipple | pa'pilliform |
| thel- | [thēl] | nipple | thel'oncus |
| later- | [latər] | side | uni'lateral |
| omphal- | [omfal] | navel | om'phalocele |

| Elements | Pronunciations | Meanings | Examples |
|---|---|---|---|
| inguin- | [ingwin] | genital area | inguino'dynia |
| dors- | [dors] | back | dorso'sacral |
| lumb- | [ləmb] | loins | lumbo'costal |
| glut- | [glūt] | buttocks | 'gluteal |
| crur- | [krūr] | leg | 'crural |
| scel- | [sei] | leg | i'sosceles |
| ped(i)-, ped- | [ped] | foot | pedi'algia |
| pod- | [päd] | foot | podarth'ritis |
| acr- | [a·kr] | extremities | acrohypo'thermy |
| mel- | [meł] | limbs | aniso'melia |

*Terminations*

| | | | |
|---|---|---|---|
| -pachynsis (pachyn/sis) | [pakinsis] | thickening | myopa'chynsis |
| -paresis (pare/sis) | [pärēsis] | weakness, partial paralysis | angiopa'resis |
| -plania (plan/ia) | [plānēə] | deviation, abnormal location | galacto'plania |

*Exercise*

Provide definitions for the following terms.

1. acromegaly ______
2. intercrural ______
3. polymastia ______
4. onychomalacia ______
5. stethoscope ______
6. trichomycosis ______
7. dactylocampsia ______
8. omphalorrhagia ______
9. bilateral ______
10. anisoscelia ______
11. trachelismus ______

12. menoplania ______________________________

13. myopachynsis ______________________________

14. microprosopia ______________________________

15. enteroparesis ______________________________

16. gynecomastic ______________________________

17. chiropodist ______________________________

18. podiatrist ______________________________

19. prosopotocia ______________________________

20. papillate ______________________________

# Chapter 14

# ABBREVIATIONS USED IN PRESCRIPTIONS AND CHARTING

The medical abbreviations contained in this chapter are derived from Latin words and phrases. They reflect an era when Latin was the common medium of communication in medical communities. The original Latin is provided to show how the abbreviations are derived. Most medical abbreviations are suspended: the first letter(s) of the Latin word(s) are used. *Post cibum* becomes p. c., *signetur* becomes sig. The abbreviation gt. uses the first letter of each syllable of the Latin *gutta*. The abbreviation ft. is an example of a contracted abbreviation: the first and last letters of the Latin word *fiat* are used. Suspended and contracted abbreviations use periods or strokes above the letter(s) to indicate their abbreviated status. Notice the difference between c. 'about' and c̄ 'with'. Abbreviations of these types occasionally indicate pluralization by doubling the last letter of the abbreviation, as in gtt. 'drops'. Arbitrary symbols are also used as abbreviations. A meaning is assigned to an arbitrary symbol, but the symbol itself may not be derived from the Latin term with which it corresponds. The abbreviation ʒ 'dram' is of this last type.

It is necessary to separate metric measurements from apothecary measurements when using these abbreviations with numbers. The quantity is written in Arabic numbers before the metric abbreviations, and in Roman numerals after apothecary measurements. 1.0 gm. is one gram; 0.250 gm. is 250 milligrams; ʒ i is one dram; gtt. ii is two drops.

| Abbreviations | Latin Sources | Meanings |
|---|---|---|
| a. c. | ante cibum | before meals |
| b. i. d. | bis in diem | twice a day |
| h. s. | hora somni | at bedtime |
| m. et n. | mane et nocte | morning and night |
| p. c. | post cibum | after meals |
| p. r. n. | pro re nata | as the occasion arises |
| q. h. | quaque hora | every hour |
| q.___h. | quaque___hora | every___hours |
| q. i. d. | quater in diem | four times a day |
| q. q. h. | quaque quarta hora | every four hours |
| quotid. | quotidie | daily |
| s. o. s. | si opus sit | if the need arises |
| stat. | statim | immediately |
| t. i. d. | ter in diem | three times a day |

| Abbreviations | Latin Sources | Meanings |
|---|---|---|
| ut dict. | ut dictum | as directed |
| aq. | aqua | water |
| aq. dest. | aqua destillata | distilled water |
| sol. | solutio | solution |
| i. m. | intra musculum | within a muscle |
| i. v. | intra venam | within a vein |
| O. D. | oculus dexter | right eye |
| O. S. | oculus sinister | left eye |
| O. U. | oculus uterque | each eye |
| p. o. | per os | orally |
| ad lib. | ad libitum | at will, freely |
| c., ca. | circa | about |
| q. l. | quantum libet | as much as desired |
| q. s. | quantum sufficiat | as much as suffices |
| rep. | repetatur | let it be repeated |
| non rep. | non repetatur | let it not be repeated |
| c̄ | cum | with |
| s̄ | sine | without |
| ad | ad | to, up to |
| d. | da | give |
| d. t. d. | dentur tales doses | let___such doses be given |
| # | | let___such doses be given |
| ft. | fiat | let there be made |
| n. b. | nota bene | note well |
| solv. | solve | dissolve |
| s̄s̄ | semis | half |
| st. | stet | let it stand |
| sum. | sume | take |
| sig. | signetur | let it be labelled |

| Abbreviations | Latin Sources | Meanings |
|---|---|---|
| *Apothecary Measurements* | | |
| cap. | capsula | capsule |
| gr. | granum | grain |
| gt. | gutta | drop |
| tab. | tabella | tablet |
| ʒ | drachma | dram |
| fʒ | fluidrachma | fluid dram |
| ℥ | uncia | ounce |
| f℥ | fluiduncia | fluid ounce |
| *Metric Measurements* | | |
| cc. | centimetrum cubicum | cubic centimeter |
| gm., Gm., G. | gramma | gram |
| mgm., mg. | milligramma | milligram |

*Exercise*

Transcribe the following prescriptions. ______________________

1. milk of magnesia ℥ i, p.o., h.s., p.r.n. ______________________
2. ferrous sulfate gr.v, t.i.d. ______________________
3. digitoxin 0.1 mgm., p.o., quotid. ______________________
4. morphine sulfate 5 mgm., i.v., q. 6 h. ______________________
5. antacid of choice 30 cc., one hour a.c., one hour p.c., h.s. ______________________
6. warm saline irrigation, O.U., m. et n. ______________________
7. tetracycline 2 Gm., i.v., q.i.d. ______________________
8. chloral hydrate 1 Gm., p.o., h.s. rep. 0.5 Gm. s.o.s. ______________________
9. heparin sodium 5000 units, i.v., stat. ______________________
10. KCl 15% sol., 10 cc., t.i.d., p.c. ______________________
11. Aq. penicillin 1,200,000 units, i.m., q. 12 h. ______________________
12. up in room c̄ eyeglasses ad lib., patch over O.S., h.s. s̄ eyeshield ______________________
13. aluminum phosphate gel ℥ s̄s̄, one hour p.c., p.r.n. ______________________

14. Multivitamin caps. xxx. Sig: cap. i quotid. ____________________
15. Neosporin eye gtt. ii., O.S., q.i.d. ____________________
16. tincture of belladonna gtt. xv c̄ aq. ℥ iv, t.i.d., a.c. ____________________
17. spiritus frumenti ℥ i, aq. dest. q.s. ad ℥ iv, sum. q.i.d. ad lib. ____________________
18. zinc oxide ointment 30 Gm., ut dict. ____________________
19. n.b. do not exceed tab. iv quotid. ____________________
20. adrenalin 0.2 cc., 1:1000 sol., ut dict. ____________________

## Chapter 15

# NUMBERS, PLURALS, COLORS

In this chapter Greek and Roman numbers are presented. It is essential that the Greek forms be kept separate from the Latin forms when these numbers are used metrically. The Latin forms yield fractions in the metric system, the Greek forms yield whole numbers. A milligram (Latin *mill(i)-*) is 1/1000 gram; a hectogram (Greek *hect(o)-*) is 100 grams.

| Elements | Pronunciations | Meanings | Examples |
|---|---|---|---|
| *Greek Numbers* | | | |
| hemi-(prefix) | [hemē, hemə] | half | 'hemitrope |
| mon- | [män] | one | mo'necious |
| prot- | [prōt] | first | pro'togynous |
| di-(prefix) | [dī] | two | 'diphyllous |
| dipl- | [di·pl] | double | diplo'gangliate |
| deuter- | [dūtər] | second | deute'roscopy |
| dich- | [dīk] | in two | di'chogamy |
| tri-(prefix) | [trī] | three | tri'morphism |
| tripl- | [tri·pl] | triple | triplo'blastic |
| tetr(a)- | [te·tr] | four | tetra'dactylous |
| pent(a)- | [pent] | five | 'pentad |
| hex(a)- | [heks] | six | 'hexapod |
| hept(a)- | [hept] | seven | 'heptode |
| oct(a)- | [äkt] | eight | 'octochord |
| enne(a)- | [enē] | nine | 'enneastyle |
| dec(a)-, dek(a)- | [dek] | ten | de'camerous |
| hect- | [hekt] | 100 | hec'tometer |
| kil- | [kil] | 1000 | 'kilogram |

| Elements | Pronunciations | Meanings | Examples |
|---|---|---|---|
| *Latin Numbers* | | | |
| semi-(prefix) | [semē] | half | semi'aerial |
| un(i)- | [yūn] | one | 'unicorn |
| prim(i)-, prim- | [prim, prīm] | first | primi'gravida |
| du-, du(i)- | [dū] | two | 'dual |
| bi-, bin-(prefix) | [bī] | two | 'bifurcate |
| second-, secund(i)- | [sekənd] | second | secundi'gravida |
| tri-(prefix) | [trī] | three | 'trident |
| terti- | [tərshē] | third | 'tertiary |
| quadr(i)-, quadr(u)- | [kwä·dr] | four | quad'rigamist |
| quinqu(e)- | [qwin·kw] | five | quinque'lateral |
| sex-(prefix), sex(i)- | [seks] | six | sex'digitate |
| sept(i)- | [sept] | seven | sep'tipara |
| oct(i)- | [äkt] | eight | 'octave |
| non(i)- | [nän] | nine | no'nipara |
| dec(i)- | [des] | ten | de'cimeter |
| cent(i)- | [sent] | 100 | 'centipede |
| mill(i)- | [mil] | 1000 | 'milligram |

Many nouns in scientific terminology still require the use of Greek and Latin endings to indicate their singular and plural forms. The italicized letters show the contrast between the singular and plural form in the examples below.

| Singular | Plural |
|---|---|
| adeno*ma* | adeno*mata* |
| antr*um* | antr*a* |
| burs*a* | burs*ae* |
| calcul*us* | calcul*i* |
| gangli*on* | gangli*a* |
| meni*nx* | meni*nges* |
| appendi*x* | appendi*ces* |
| neuro*sis* | neuro*ses* |

| Elements | Pronunciations | Meanings | Examples |
|---|---|---|---|
| *Colors* | | | |
| melan- | [melən] | black | melan'oma |
| leuk- | [lūk] | white | leuko'rrhea |
| poli- | [pōlē] | gray | poliomye'litis |
| glauc-, glauk- | [glawk] | gray-green | glau'comatous |
| erythr- | [erith·r] | red | e'rythrocyte |
| chlor- | [klor] | green | chlor'opia |
| cyan- | [sīən] | blue | cyan'osis |
| xanth- | [zanth] | yellow | xantho'dontous |
| *alb-, albid- | [albid] | white | albi'duria |
| *rub(e)-, rubr- | [rūb] | red | 'rubric |

*Exercise*

Provide definitions for the following terms.

1. chloremia __________
2. cyanodermia __________
3. sexdigital __________
4. hemicardia __________
5. monochromatic __________
6. tripod __________
7. hemigastrectomy __________
8. pentamerous __________
9. unilateral __________
10. bigamy __________

Provide a plural form corresponding to each of the singular forms given below.

1. fibroma __________
2. addendum __________
3. antenna __________
4. ovum __________
5. phalanx __________
6. bacillus __________

7. axis ______________________________
8. diagnosis ______________________________
9. stoma ______________________________
10. alumnus ______________________________

# Chapter 16

# MISCELLANEOUS FORMS, DIMINUTIVES

| Elements | Pronunciations | Meanings | Examples |
|---|---|---|---|
| *Base Forms* | | | |
| adelph- | [adelf] | brother | adel'phogamy |
| cry- | [krī] | cold | cryes'thesia |
| cut(i)-, cutan- | [kyūtān] | skin | cu'taneous |
| dorm(i)- | [dorm] | sleep | predor'mition |
| ger-, geront- | [jeränt] | old, old person | geron'topia |
| hist- | [hist] | tissue | 'histotribe |
| in- | [in] | fiber | inoscle'rosis |
| luc(i)- | [lūs] | light | trans'lucent |
| lun- | [lūn] | moon | semi'lunar |
| macul- | [makyūl] | spot | macu'lation |
| pariet- | [pərīət] | wall | pa'rietal |
| path- | [pəthē] | feeling | an'tipathy |
| sanguin-, sangu(i)- | [saŋ·gw] | blood | san'guicolous |
| syring- | [siriŋ·g] | tube, pipe | syringo'myelocele |
| thanat- | [thanət] | death | thanato'phobia |
| thec- | [thēk] | sheath, case | oo'theca |
| archae-, arche- | [ärkē] | ancient | archae'ologist |
| palae-, pale- | [pālē] | old, ancient | paleo'lithic |
| magn- | [mag·n] | large | 'magnify |
| parv(i)- | [parv] | small | parvi'cellular |
| mult(i)- | [mult] | much, many | multi'cuspidate |
| plur(i)- | [plūr] | many, more | pluri'gravida |
| null(i)- | [nəl] | none, no | 'nullify |
| cac-, kak- | [kak] | bad | caco'geusia |
| idi- | [idē] | one's own, peculiar | idio'genic |

| Elements | Pronunciations | Meanings | Examples |
|---|---|---|---|
| plat(y)- | [plat] | flat | platy'pelvic |
| stere- | [sterē] | solid | 'stereoscope |
| sicc- | [sik] | dry | 'desiccate |
| furc- | [fərk] | forked | bifur'cation |
| cau-, caus- | [kos] | burn | cau'salgia |
| cid- | [sid] | fall | pro'ciduous |
| gno- | [g·no] | know | stereog'nosis |
| mis- | [mis] | hate | miso'pedia |
| mne- | [m·nē] | remember | hypom'nesia |
| phan- | [fān] | show, appear | meno'phania |

*Suffix*

| | | | |
|---|---|---|---|
| -uous | [yūus] | pertaining to | de'ciduous |

*Diminutive Suffixes*

| | | | |
|---|---|---|---|
| -cule, -cle | [kəl] | | 'cuticle |
| -ellum | [eləm] | | fla'gellum |
| -il | [il] | | myo'fibril |
| -isk, -iscus | [isk] | | 'asterisk |
| -ium, -ion | [ēəm] | | pseudo'podium |
| -ule, -ole | [ol] | | 'bronchiole |

Diminutive suffixes all imply the physical smallness of the elements which precede them. Thus their usual meaning is 'little'.

*Terminations*

| | | | |
|---|---|---|---|
| -helcosis, -elcosis (helc/o/sis) | [elkōsis] | ulceration | enterel'cosis |
| -atresia (a/tre/sia) | [atrēzēə] | imperforation | urethra'tresia |
| -spasm (spas/m) | [spasəm] | spasm | 'cardiospasm |

| Elements | Pronunciations | Meanings | Examples |
|---|---|---|---|
| -lepsy (leps/y) | [lepsē] | seizure | 'hypnolepsy |
| -cenosis (cen/o/sis) | [senōsis] | evacuation | hydrocen'osis |
| -oncus (onc/us) | [onkus] | tumor | oste'oncus |
| -aphia (aph/ia) | [āfēə] | touch | hyper'aphia |
| -osmia (osm/ia) | [osmēə] | smell | hy'posmia |
| -orexia (orex/ia) | [ōreksēə] | appetite | ano'rexia |

The Greek adjective *idios* means private, personal, one's own, precisely its meaning in medical and scientific terminology. It is not until medieval times that the word, passing through Latin, acquired the meaning of ignorant person and eventually of one who is mentally deficient. Also the original meaning of the Greek word *syrinx* was shepherd's pipe. Obviously medicine and science have modified this term to apply to tubes and pipes sharing the same shape as a shepherd's pipe.

*Exercise*

Provide definitions for the following terms.

1. cacosmia ____________________
2. subcutaneous ____________________
3. cryotherapy ____________________
4. ossicle ____________________
5. prognosis ____________________
6. histolysis ____________________
7. idiopathic ____________________
8. multilateral ____________________
9. thanatophobia ____________________
10. colpatresia ____________________
11. radicle ____________________
12. gastrohelcosis ____________________
13. polyadelphous ____________________
14. venule ____________________

15. gerontology ______________________________________________

16. capitellum ______________________________________________

17. podium ______________________________________________

18. auricle ______________________________________________

19. syringoid ______________________________________________

20. arteriole ______________________________________________

## Chapter 17

# GENERAL BIOLOGICAL-ZOOLOGICAL FORMS

| Elements | Pronunciations | Meanings | Examples |
|---|---|---|---|
| *Prefixes* | | | |
| in-, im-, ir-, il- | [in] | into, on | in'seminate |
| in-, im-, ir-, il- | [im] | not, without | im'maculate |
| *Base Forms* | | | |
| anth- | [anth] | flower | mo'nanthous |
| bry- | [brī] | moss | 'bryophyte |
| carp- | [kärp] | fruit | carpo'genic |
| cortic- | [kortik] | bark, cortex | 'corticate |
| dendr- | [den·dr] | tree | 'dendroid |
| foli- | [fōlē] | leaf | pluri'foliate |
| gymn- | [jim·n] | naked, uncovered | gymno'carpous |
| phyc- | [fīk] | algae, seaweed | phy'cology |
| phyll- | [fil] | leaf | phyl'lophagous |
| ram(i)- | [ram] | branch | 'ramiform |
| branchi- | [braŋ·kē] | gill | 'branchiopod |
| caud- | [kod] | tail | 'caudad |
| helminth- | [helminth] | worm | helmin'thiasis |
| herpet- | [herpit] | snake, reptile | herpe'tology |
| hipp- | [hip] | horse | 'hippodrome |
| ichthy- | [ikthē] | fish | ichthy'osis |
| ornith-, ornis- | [ornith] | bird | 'ornithoid |
| pter- | [ter] | wing, fin | ptero'dactyl |
| penn- | [pen] | feather | 'pennate |

| Elements | Pronunciations | Meanings | Examples |
|---|---|---|---|
| ventr-, ventr(i)- | [ven·tr] | stomach, belly | ventro'dorsal |
| verm(i)- | [verm] | worm | 'vermiform |
| zo- | [zō] | animal, living being | zoo'genic |
| carn(i)- | [kärn] | flesh | 'carnivore |
| col- | [kol] | inhabitant | san'guicolous |
| corp-, corpor- | [korpər] | body | in'corporate |
| de- | [də, dē] | bind | 'syndesis |
| ec-, oec-, oik- | [ēk] | house, environment | e'cology |
| fil- | [fil] | thread | 'filiform |
| mit- | [mīt] | thread | mito'chondria |
| morph- | [morf] | form | homo'morphous |
| nomin-, nom- | [nämən, nōm] | name | 'nominate |
| onym-, onom- | [änəm] | name | pseu'donymous |
| pil(i)- | [pil] | hair | pi'liferous |
| phyl- | [fīl] | race | phylo'genic |
| ret-, reticul- | [retikyūl] | network | re'ticulate |
| sect- | [sekt] | cut | 'dissect |
| sit- | [sīt] | food | si'tology |
| tax- | [taks] | arrange | tax'onomy |
| trep-, trop- | [trep, träp] | turn | photo'tropic |
| troph- | [träf] | nourish | 'trophoblast |
| viv(i)- | [vīv, viv] | alive | vi'viparous |
| vor- | [vər] | eat | car'nivorous |
| xen- | [zen] | foreign, host | xe'nogamy |

*Terminations*

| | | | |
|---|---|---|---|
| -(a)tion | [(ā)shən] | action, condition | defoli'ation |

When the prefix de- is used with the termination -(a)tion the two elements frequently mean 'removal'.

| | | | |
|---|---|---|---|
| -be | | living organism | 'aerobe |
| -facient | [fāshənt] | producing | rube'facient |

| Elements | Pronunciations | Meanings | Examples |
|---|---|---|---|
| -auxe (aux/e) | [awksē] | increase, enlargement | hepat'auxe |
| -cide (cid/e) | [sīd] | killing agent | 'vermicide |
| -nomy (nom/y) | [nomē] | regulation | e'conomy |
| -plasia (plas/ia) | [plāzēə] | formation | dys'plasia |
| -taxy (tax/y) | [taksē] | arrangement | phyllo'taxy |

*Exercise*

Provide definitions for the following terms.

1. anthophilous __________
2. decorticate __________
3. dendrochronology __________
4. mastauxe __________
5. xenophobia __________
6. autotrophic __________
7. anisopterous __________
8. anonymous __________
9. dehydration __________
10. lactivorous __________
11. febrifacient __________
12. biramose __________
13. retiform __________
14. depilation __________
15. vivisect __________
16. ichthyology __________
17. reticule __________
18. revivify __________
19. allomorphic __________
20. foliose __________

# Chapter 18

# LATIN IN ENGLISH USAGE

The English language contains many Latin words, phrases, and abbreviations from various fields outside medicine and science. What follows is an arbitrary list of Latin items, primarily legal and literary, and their general connotations.

| | |
|---|---|
| caveat emptor | let the buyer beware |
| amicus curiae | friend of the court; legal advisor to a court |
| obiter dictum | incidental remark |
| ad litem | for the suit |
| licet | it is allowed |
| mandamus | we command; writ demanding performance of an official act |
| nolo contendere | I do not wish to contest; plea declaring no defense will be made, but no guilt is admitted |
| quid pro quo | one thing for another, substitute |
| quo warranto | by what authority; writ questioning by what right an office or privilege is held |
| prima facie | on first sight |
| bona fide | in good faith |
| de facto | actually |
| de jure | legally |
| ex parte | one sided, in the interest of one side |
| ex post facto | retroactive, retrospective |
| habeas corpus | writ questioning the legality of a person's restraint |
| ipso facto | by the very nature of the case |
| sine die | without a day (appointed) |
| sine qua non | prerequisite |
| per diem | by the day |
| per annum | by the year |
| ex cathedra | from the chair; authoritative pronouncement |
| in loco parentis | in the place of a parent |

| | |
|---|---|
| magna cum laude | with great praise |
| summa cum laude | with greatest praise |
| terminus ad quem | latest possible date; destination |
| terminus a quo | earliest possible date; point of origin |
| ad hoc | for this (case only) |
| ad infinitum | without end |
| a fortiori | all the more |
| a posteriori | effect to cause, inductively |
| a priori | cause to effect, deductively |
| ceteris paribus | other things being equal |
| corpus | body, collection of writings |
| ex officio | by virtue of office |
| ex tempore | unrehearsed |
| pro tempore | for the time (being) |
| gratis | freely |
| in situ | in the original position |
| inter alia | among other things |
| in toto | entirely |
| modus operandi | manner of acting |
| modus vivendi | manner of living |
| mutatis mutandis | necessary changes having been made |
| non sequitur | illogical statement |
| opus | work, book |
| per se | by itself, intrinsically |
| post mortem | after death |
| pro forma | for the sake of form |
| qua | as |
| re | regarding |
| seriatim | in order |
| status quo | existing condition |
| sub rosa | secretly |
| sui generis | unique |

| Abbreviations | Sources | Meanings |
|---|---|---|
| loc. cit. | loco citato | in the place cited |
| op. cit. | opere citato | in the work cited |
| ibid. | ibidem | the same (place) |
| cf. | confer | compare |
| vid. | vide | see |
| e. g. | exempli gratia | for example |
| i. e. | id est | that is |
| seq. | sequente | following |
| et al. | et alii | and others |
| etc. | et cetera | and the rest |
| vs. | versus | against |
| q. e. d. | quod erat demonstrandum | proof |

# REVIEW B

Review B consists of fifty terms which concentrate on the elements introduced in the last nine chapters. Write the definitions for these terms in the spaces provided and then check your answers by consulting the indices in the back of the text.

acrohyperhidrosis ______

amniorrhexis ______

aniridia ______

auriform ______

bicornuous ______

blepharopachynsis ______

chiromegaly ______

chloropia ______

cryptomenorrhea

dacryelcosis

gynecomastia

heminephrectomy

hepatomelanosis

hexadactylism

histonomy

innominate

macroscelia

melanomata

metrostaxis

monocyesis

myringoscope

omentosplenopexy

oophorauxe

ophthalmogyric

orthodontia

oscheoplasty

otoneurasthenia

pachyonychia

palaeolithic

pericolpitis

phacoplania

phalloncus

primipara

pteropod

quadrifoliate

serosanguineous

spermatoschesis

superfetation

syringosystrophy

tenontothecitis

thoracocentesis

tocology

triorchidism

ulorrhea

uniocular

uranoschisis

uvulaptosis

vivisection

xanthuria

xerophobia

# INDEX OF PREFIXES

-A-

| | |
|---|---|
| a-, an- | not, without |
| a-, ab-, abs- | from, away from |
| ad- | to, toward, near |
| ambi- | both |
| amphi-, ampho- | both, on both sides |
| ana- | up, again |
| ante- | before, in front |
| anti- | against |
| apo- | from, away |

-C-

| | |
|---|---|
| cata- | down, very |
| circum- | around |
| con-, com-, col- | with together, completely |
| contra-, contro- | opposite, against |

-D-

| | |
|---|---|
| de- | down, away |
| dia- | through, across |
| dis-, dif-, di- | apart |
| dys- | poor, painful |

-E-

| | |
|---|---|
| ec-, ex- | out |
| ecto-, exo- | outer, outside |
| en-, em-, el- | in, into |
| endo-, ento- | inner, inside |
| epi- | upon, over |

| | |
|---|---|
| eso- | inward |
| eu- | well, good |
| extra-, extro- | outside, beyond |

-H-

| | |
|---|---|
| hyper- | excessive |
| hypo- | below, deficient |

-I-

| | |
|---|---|
| in-, im-, ir-, il- | not, without |
| in-, im-, ir-, il- | on, into |
| infra- | below |
| inter- | between, among |
| intra-, intro- | within |

-J-

| | |
|---|---|
| juxta- | close to |

-M-

| | |
|---|---|
| meta- | after, changed |

-P-

| | |
|---|---|
| pan- | all, complete |
| para- | beside, abnormal |
| per- | through, completely |
| peri- | around |
| post- | after, behind |
| pre- | before |
| pro- | forward |
| pros- | toward, in addition |

-R-

| | |
|---|---|
| re- | back, again |
| retro- | backward |

-S-

| | |
|---|---|
| sub-, sup-, suc- | under |
| super- | over, excessive |
| supra- | above |
| syn-, sym-, syl- | with, together |

-T-

| | |
|---|---|
| tele- | afar, at a distance |
| trans- | across |

-U-

| | |
|---|---|
| ultra- | beyond |

# INDEX OF SUFFIXES AND TERMINATIONS

-A-

| | |
|---|---|
| -ac | pertaining to |
| -ad | toward, in the direction of |
| -agogue | agent inducing flow |
| -al | pertaining to |
| -algia | pain |
| -aphia | touch |
| -ar | pertaining to |
| -ary | pertaining to |
| -ase | enzyme |
| -asthenia | condition of no strength (weakness) |
| -ate | to make |
| -ate | having |
| -atresia | imperforation |
| -atrophy | no development (absence of development) |
| -auxe | increase, enlargement |

-B-

| | |
|---|---|
| -be | living organism |
| -blast | embryonic cell |

-C-

| | |
|---|---|
| -campsia | bending, curvature |
| -cele | hernia(tion), swelling |
| -cenosis | evacuation |
| -centesis | surgical puncture |
| -chezia | defecation |
| -cide | killing agent |
| -clasis, -clasia | fracture |
| -clysis | irrigation, washing |
| -cule, -cle | little |

| | |
|---|---|
| -cyesis | pregnancy |
| -cyte | cell |

-E-

| | |
|---|---|
| -e | instrument |
| -eal | pertaining to |
| -ectasis, -ectasia | dilatation, stretching |
| -ectomy | excision, surgical removal |
| -ectopy, -ectopia | displacement |
| -edema | swelling |
| -ellum | little |
| -emesis | vomiting |
| -emia | blood condition |
| -emphraxis | obstruction |
| -esthesia | sensitivity, perception |
| -eurynter | dilator |

-F-

| | |
|---|---|
| -facient | producing |
| -ferous, -feric | bearing, carrying |
| -form | having the shape of |
| -fy | to make |

-G-

| | |
|---|---|
| -genous, -genic | causing, caused by |
| -geusia | taste |
| -gram | a record(ing) |
| -graphy | state of recording |
| -gravida | a woman who is pregnant |

H

| | |
|---|---|
| -helocosis, -elcosis | ulceration |

## -I-

| | |
|---|---|
| -ia | condition of |
| -iasis | presence of, infestation |
| -ic | pertaining to |
| -ician | specialist in |
| -ics | system |
| -il | little |
| -in, ine | substance |
| -isk, -iscus | little |
| -ism | state of, condition of |
| -ismus | spasm |
| -ist | one who (specializes in) |
| -itis | inflammation |
| -ium, -ion | little |
| -ize | to make |

## -K-

| | |
|---|---|
| -kinesis, -kinesia | movement |

## -L-

| | |
|---|---|
| -lepsy | seizure |
| -lith | stone, calculus |
| -logy | study |
| -lysis | dissolution, destruction |

## -M-

| | |
|---|---|
| -malacia | softening |
| -megaly | enlargement |
| -mere, -mer | part |
| -meter | instrument to measure |
| -metry | measurement |

-N-

| | |
|---|---|
| -necrosis | death, dead condition |
| -nomy | regulation |

-O-

| | |
|---|---|
| -odynia | pain |
| -oid | resembling, like |
| -oma | tumor |
| -omatosis | abnormal condition of tumors |
| -omatous | pertaining to tumors |
| -oncus | tumor |
| -opia, -opsia | vision |
| -orexia | appetite |
| -ose | pertaining to, full of |
| -osis | abnormal condition |
| -osmia | smell |
| -osteosis, -ostosis | ossification, calcification |
| -ous | pertaining to |

-P-

| | |
|---|---|
| -pachynsis | thickening |
| -para | a woman who has given birth |
| -paresis | weakness, partial paralysis |
| -pathy | a disease |
| -penia | deficiency |
| -pepsia | digestion |
| -pexy | fixation |
| -philia | affinity, love |
| -physis | growing |
| -phyte | growth |
| -piesis | pressure |
| -plania | deviation, abnormal location |
| -plasia | formation |

| | |
|---|---|
| -plasty | surgical repair |
| -plegia | paralysis, stroke |
| -pnea | breathing |
| -poiesis | production, formation |
| -ptosis | prolapse, sagging |

-R-

| | |
|---|---|
| -rrhagia | hemorrhage |
| -rrhaphy | suture |
| -rrhea | flow |
| -rrhexis | rupture |

-S-

| | |
|---|---|
| -schesis, -schesia | suppression, retention |
| -schisis | splitting |
| -sclerosis | hardening |
| -scope | instrument for examining |
| -scopy | examination |
| -sepsis | infection |
| -sis, -sia | condition of |
| -spasm | spasm |
| -stalsis, -stole | contraction |
| -stasis | stopping, controlling |
| -stat | instrument for stopping |
| -staxis | dripping, oozing |
| -stenosis | narrowing |
| -sthenia | strength |
| -stomy | creation of (new) opening |

-T-

| | |
|---|---|
| -t | instrument |
| -taxy | arrangement |
| -therapy | treatment |
| -thesis | putting, placing |
| -tic | pertaining to |

| | |
|---|---|
| -(a)tion | action, condition |
| -tome | instrument to cut |
| -tomy | incision |
| -tribe, -trite | instrument for crushing |
| -tripsy | surgical crushing |
| -trophy, -trophia | development, nourishment |

-U-

| | |
|---|---|
| -ule, -ole | little |
| -uous | pertaining to |
| -uria | urine condition |

-Y-

| | |
|---|---|
| -y | state of |

# INDEX OF BASE FORMS

-A-

| | |
|---|---|
| abdomin- | abdomen |
| acet-, acet(i)- | acid, vinegar |
| acou-, acu- | hear |
| acr- | extremities |
| acromi- | acromium |
| actin- | ray, x ray |
| adamantin-, adamant- | enamel |
| adelph- | brother |
| aden- | gland |
| adenoid- | adenoid |
| adip- | (animal) fat |
| aer- | air, gas |
| alb-, albid- | white |
| all- | other, different |
| alveol- | tooth socket |
| ambl(y)- | dull |
| amel- | enamel |
| amni- | amnion, amniotic fluid |
| amyl- | starch |
| an- | anus |
| andr- | man (male) |
| angi- | vessel |
| anth- | flower |
| anthrop- | human being, man |
| antr- | cavity |
| aort- | aorta |
| apic- | apex, tip |
| append-, appendic- | appendix |

| | |
|---|---|
| aqu(e)-, aqu(a)- | water |
| archae-, arche- | ancient |
| argent(i)-, argent- | silver |
| arteri- | artery |
| arthr- | joint |
| articul- | joint |
| astr- | star, star-shaped |
| astragal- | astragalus |
| atel- | incomplete, imperfect |
| atri- | atrium |
| audi-, audit- | hear |
| aur(i)-, aur- | gold |
| aur(i)-, aur- | ear |
| auricul- | auricle |
| aut- | self, one's own |
| axill- | armpit |

-B-

| | |
|---|---|
| balan- | glans penis |
| bar- | weight, pressure |
| bar(y)- | heavy |
| bi- | life, living |
| bi-, bin- | two |
| blast- | embryonic cell |
| blenn- | mucus |
| blep- | vision |
| blephar- | eyelid |
| brachi- | arm |
| brach(y)- | short |
| brad(y)- | slow |
| branchi- | gill |
| bromat- | food |
| bronch-, bronchi- | bronchus |

| | |
|---|---|
| bronchiol- | bronchiole |
| bry- | moss |
| bucc- | cheek |
| burs- | bursa |

-C-

| | |
|---|---|
| cac-, kak- | bad |
| calcane- | calcaneum (calcaneus) |
| capillar- | capillary |
| capit-, -cipit- | head |
| carcin- | cancer |
| cardi- | heart |
| carn(i)- | flesh |
| carp- | carpus |
| carp- | fruit |
| cau-, caus- | burn |
| caud- | tail |
| cec- | cecum |
| celi- | abdominal cavity |
| cent(i)- | 100 |
| cephal- | head |
| cerebell- | cerebellum |
| cerebr- | cerebrum |
| cervic- | cervix, neck |
| cheil- | lip |
| chir-, cheir- | hand |
| chlor- | green |
| chol(e)-, chol- | bile |
| cholecyst- | gallbladder |
| choledoch- | (common) bile duct |
| chondr- | cartilage |
| chord- | (vocal) cord |
| choroid- | choroid |

| | |
|---|---|
| chromat-, chrom- | color |
| chron- | time |
| chrys- | gold |
| cicatric- | scar |
| cid- | fall |
| cili- | eyelash |
| clavicul- | clavicle |
| coccyg- | coccyx |
| cochle- | cochlea |
| col- | inhabitant |
| col-, colon- | colon, large intestine |
| coll- | glue, gelatin |
| colp- | vagina |
| condyl- | condyle |
| coni- | dust |
| conjunctiv- | conjunctiva |
| copr- | excrement |
| cor-, core- | pupil |
| corne- | cornea |
| corn(i)-, corn(u)- | horn |
| corp-, corpor- | body |
| cortic- | bark, cortex |
| cost- | rib |
| cox- | hip joint |
| crani- | skull |
| crin- | secrete |
| crot- | pulse beat |
| crur- | leg |
| cry- | cold |
| crypt- | hidden |
| cuspid- | point |
| cut-, cutan- | skin |
| cyan- | blue |

| | |
|---|---|
| cycl- | ciliary body |
| cyst- | bladder, sac |
| cyt- | cell |

-D-

| | |
|---|---|
| dacry- | tear, tear duct |
| dactyl- | finger, toe |
| de- | bind |
| dec(a)-, dek(a)- | ten |
| dec(i)- | ten |
| dem- | people, country |
| dendr- | tree |
| dent(i)-, dent- | tooth |
| dentin- | dentin |
| dermat-, derm- | skin |
| desm- | ligament |
| deuter- | second |
| dextr- | right |
| di- | two |
| dich- | in two |
| digit- | finger, toe |
| dipl- | double |
| dips- | thirst |
| dist- | farthest |
| doch- | duct |
| dolich- | long |
| dorm(i)- | sleep |
| dors- | back |
| drom- | running, course |
| du-, du(i)- | two |
| duoden- | duodenum |
| dyn-, dynam- | power |

-E-

| | |
|---|---|
| ec-, oec-, oik- | house, environment |
| electr- | electricity |
| encephal- | brain |
| enne(a)- | nine |
| enter- | small intestine |
| epididym- | epididymis |
| epiglottid-, epiglott- | epiglottis |
| epipl- | omentum |
| erythr- | red |
| esophag- | esophagus |
| eti- | cause |
| eur(y)- | wide |
| eustach- | eustachian tube |

-F-

| | |
|---|---|
| faci- | face |
| fec-, fecal- | excrement |
| femor- | femur |
| fenestr- | window |
| ferr(i)-, ferr- | iron |
| fet- | fetus |
| fibr- | fiber |
| fibul- | fibula |
| fil- | thread |
| foli- | leaf |
| fren- | frenum, frenulum |
| furc- | forked |

-G-

| | |
|---|---|
| galact- | milk |
| gam- | marriage |
| gangli-, ganglion- | ganglion |

| | |
|---|---|
| gastr- | stomach |
| ge- | earth |
| ger-, geront- | old, old person |
| gingiv- | gums |
| glauc-, glauk- | gray-green |
| globul- | globule, corpuscle |
| glomerul- | glomerulus |
| gloss- | tongue |
| glott- | glottis |
| glut- | buttocks |
| glyc-, gluc- | sugar |
| gnath- | jaw |
| gno- | know |
| gymn- | naked, uncovered |
| gyn-, gynec- | women (female) |
| gyr- | orbit, circle |

-H-

| | |
|---|---|
| hal(i)-, hal- | salt |
| hect- | 100 |
| heli- | sun |
| helminth- | worm |
| hem-, hemat- | blood |
| hemi- | half |
| hepat- | liver |
| hept(a)- | seven |
| herpet- | snake, reptile |
| heter- | other, different |
| hex(a)- | six |
| hidr- | sweat |
| hipp- | horse |
| hist- | tissue |
| hom- | same |

| | |
|---|---|
| home- | similar |
| humer- | humerus |
| hyal- | glass |
| hydr- | water, fluid |
| hygr- | moisture |
| hypn- | sleep |
| hyster- | uterus |

-I-

| | |
|---|---|
| iatr- | healing |
| ichthy- | fish |
| idi- | one's own, peculiar |
| ile- | ileum |
| ili- | ilium |
| in- | fiber |
| incud- | incus |
| inguin- | genital area |
| ir-, irid- | iris |
| is- | equal |
| ischi- | ischium |

-J-

| | |
|---|---|
| jejun- | jejunum |

-K-

| | |
|---|---|
| kary- | nucleus |
| kerat- | horn |
| kerat- | cornea |
| kil- | 1000 |
| kym- | wave |

## -L-

| | |
|---|---|
| labi- | lip |
| labyrinth- | labyrinth |
| lacrim- | tear, tear duct |
| lact-, lact(i)- | milk |
| lapar- | abdominal wall |
| laryng- | larynx |
| later- | side |
| lei- | smooth |
| lent-, lent(i)- | lens |
| lenticul- | lens |
| lept- | thin, delicate |
| leuk- | white |
| lingu- | tongue |
| lip- | fat |
| lith- | stone, calculus |
| log- | word, understanding |
| luc(i)- | light |
| lumb- | loins |
| lun- | moon |
| lymph- | lymph |

## -M-

| | |
|---|---|
| macr- | large |
| macul- | spot |
| magn- | large |
| malle- | malleus |
| mamm(i)-, mamm- | breast |
| mandibul- | mandible |
| manu- | hand |
| mast-, maz- | breast |
| mastoid- | mastoid process |
| maxill- | maxilla |
| meat- | opening, meatus, passage |

| | |
|---|---|
| medi- | middle |
| megal-, meg(a)- | large |
| mel- | limbs |
| melan- | black |
| men- | menses, menstruation |
| mening- | meninges |
| ment- | chin |
| mer- | part |
| mes-, mesi- | middle |
| metr- | uterus |
| micr- | small |
| mill(i)- | 1000 |
| mis- | hate |
| mit- | thread |
| mne- | remember |
| mon- | one |
| morph- | form |
| muc-, muc(i)- | mucus, mucous membrane |
| mult(i)- | much, many |
| my- | muscle |
| myc-, mycet- | fungus |
| myel- | spinal cord, bone marrow |
| myring- | tympanic membrane |
| myx- | mucus |

-N-

| | |
|---|---|
| nar(i)- | nostril |
| nas-, nas(i)- | nose |
| ne- | new |
| nephr- | kidney |
| nerv(i)- | nerve |
| neur- | nerve |
| nomin-, nom- | name |

| | |
|---|---|
| non(i)- | nine |
| null(i)- | none, no |
| nyct- | night |

-O-

| | |
|---|---|
| o- | ovum, egg |
| oct(a)- | eight |
| oct(i)- | eight |
| ocul- | eye |
| od-, hod- | road, way |
| odont- | tooth |
| ole- | oil |
| olig- | little, few |
| om- | shoulder |
| oment- | omentum |
| omphal- | navel |
| onych- | nail |
| onym-, onom- | name |
| oophor- | ovary |
| ophthalm- | eye |
| opt- | vision |
| or- | mouth |
| orchi-, orchid- | testicle |
| ornith-, ornis- | bird |
| orth- | straight |
| osche- | scrotum |
| oste- | bone |
| ot- | ear |
| ov(i)-, ov- | ovum, egg |

-P-

| | |
|---|---|
| pach(y)- | thick |
| palae-, pale- | old, ancient |

| | |
|---|---|
| palat- | (hard) palate |
| palpebr- | eyelid |
| pancreat- | pancreas |
| pant- | all, complete |
| papill- | nipple |
| par- | give birth |
| pariet- | wall |
| parv(i)- | small |
| patell- | patella |
| path- | disease, feeling |
| pector- | chest |
| ped- | child |
| ped(i)-, ped- | foot |
| pelv(i)-, pelv-, pelvi- | pelvis |
| pen-, pen(i)- | penis |
| penn- | feather |
| pent(a)- | five |
| peritone-, periton- | peritoneum |
| pha-, phas-, phem- | speak |
| phac- | lens |
| phag- | eat, swallow |
| phalang- | phalanges |
| phall- | penis |
| phan- | show, appear |
| pharmac- | drug |
| pharyng- | pharynx |
| phil- | love |
| phleb- | vein |
| phob- | fear |
| phon- | sound, voice |
| phot- | light |
| phren- | diaphragm |
| phyc- | algae, seaweed |

| | |
|---|---|
| phyl- | race |
| phyll- | leaf |
| pil(i)- | hair |
| pinn- | pinna |
| plasm- | plasma |
| plat(y)- | flat |
| pleur- | pleura |
| plur(i)- | many, more |
| pne- | breathe |
| pneum- | air, lung |
| pneumat- | air, gas |
| pneumon- | lung |
| pod- | foot |
| poli- | gray (matter) |
| pol(y)- | many, much |
| prim(i)-, prim- | first |
| proct- | anus and rectum |
| prosop- | face |
| prostat- | prostate gland |
| prot- | first |
| proxim- | nearest |
| pseud- | false |
| psych- | mind, soul |
| pter- | wing, fin |
| ptyal- | saliva |
| pub-, pubi- | pubis |
| pulm-, pulmon- | lung |
| puls(i)-, puls- | pulse |
| pupill- | pupil |
| py- | pus |
| pyel- | renal pelvis |
| pylor- | pylorus |
| pyr-, pyret- | fire, fever |

-Q-

| | |
|---|---|
| quadr(u)-, quadr(i)- | four |
| quinqu(e)- | five |

-R-

| | |
|---|---|
| rachi-, rach(i)- | spine |
| radi- | ray, x ray |
| radi- | radius |
| radic-, radicul- | root |
| ram(i)- | branch |
| rect- | rectum |
| ren-, ren(i)- | kidney |
| ret-, reticul- | network |
| retin- | retina |
| rhin- | nose |
| rhiz- | root |
| rub(e)-, rubr- | red |

-S-

| | |
|---|---|
| sacchar- | sugar |
| sacr- | sacrum |
| sal(i)- | salt |
| salping- | fallopian tube |
| sanguin-, sangu(i)- | blood |
| sarc- | flesh |
| scapul- | scapula |
| scel- | leg |
| schiz-, schist- | split |
| scler- | sclera |
| scoli- | curved, bent |
| scrot- | scrotum |
| seb-, seb(i)- | tallow, grease |
| second-, secund(i)- | second |

| | |
|---|---|
| sect- | cut |
| semi- | half |
| semin- | semen |
| sept-, sept(i)- | septum |
| sept(i)- | seven |
| ser- | serum |
| sex-, sex(i)- | six |
| sial- | saliva |
| sicc- | dry |
| sigmoid- | sigmoid flexure |
| sinistr- | left |
| sin-, sinus- | sinus |
| sit- | food |
| som-, somat- | body |
| sperm-, spermat- | sperm, seed |
| sphygm- | pulse |
| spin- | spine |
| splanchn- | internal organs |
| splen- | spleen |
| spondyl- | vertebra(e) |
| squam- | scale, flake |
| sta- | stop, control |
| staped- | stapes |
| staphyl- | soft palate |
| steat-, stear- | tallow |
| stell- | star, star-shaped |
| sten- | narrow |
| stere- | solid |
| stern- | sternum |
| steth- | chest |
| sthen- | strength |
| stigmat- | mark, focus point |
| stom-, stomat- | mouth |

| | |
|---|---|
| supercili- | eyebrow |
| synovi- | synovial fluid, synovial membrane |
| syring- | tube, pipe |

-T-

| | |
|---|---|
| tach(y)- | rapid, fast |
| tal- | talus |
| tars- | tarsus |
| tax- | arrange |
| ten-, tenont- | tendon |
| tend-, tendin- | tendon |
| terti- | third |
| test-, test(i)- | testicle |
| tetr(a)- | four |
| thanat- | death |
| thec- | sheath, case |
| thel- | nipple |
| therm- | heat |
| thorac- | thorax, chest |
| thromb- | clot |
| tibi- | tibia |
| toc- | childbirth |
| ton- | tension |
| tonsill- | tonsil |
| top- | place |
| tox-, tox(i)- | poison |
| trache- | trachea |
| trachel- | neck, cervix |
| trach(y)- | rough |
| trep-, trop- | turn |
| tri- | three |
| trich- | hair |
| tripl- | triple |

| | |
|---|---|
| troph- | nourish |
| tuss- | cough |
| tympan- | tympanum |
| typhl- | cecum |

-U-

| | |
|---|---|
| ul- | gum |
| uln- | ulna |
| un(i)- | one |
| ur- | urine |
| uranisc-, uran- | (hard) palate |
| ureter- | ureter |
| urethr- | urethra |
| uter- | uterus |
| utricul- | utricle |
| uve- | uveal tract |
| uvul- | uvula |

-V-

| | |
|---|---|
| vagin- | vagina |
| vas- | vas deferens |
| vascul- | vessel |
| vel- | velum |
| ven- | vein |
| ventr-, ventr(i)- | stomach, belly |
| ventricul- | ventricle |
| verm(i)- | worm |
| vertebr- | vertebra(e) |
| vesic- | bladder, sac |
| vestibul- | vestibule |
| viscer- | internal organs |
| vitr-, vitr(i)- | glass |
| viv(i)- | alive |
| vor- | eat |

-X-

| | |
|---|---|
| xanth- | yellow |
| xen- | foreign, host |
| xer- | dry |

-Z-

| | |
|---|---|
| zo- | animal, living being |

# ANSWERS

Answers are given only for terms to be completed or provided.

Chapter 1

1. autonomous
2. megalocardia
3. pseudonym
4. endotracheal
5. chronometer
6. sigmoidoscope
7. tonsillectomy
8. enterostenosis
9. atelomyelia
10. pediatric

Chapter 2

1. bradypepsia
2. heliotropic
3. suprarenal
4. radiotherapist
5. cytoid
6. aphasia
7. craniomalacia
8. osteotome
9. heteromorphic
10. hematolysis

Chapter 3

1. amylemia
2. hydrocephalic
3. antipyretic
4. haloid
5. mycomyringitis
6. galactin
7. pyocele
8. cephalad
9. cholepoiesis
10. blennorrhea

Chapter 4

1. antithrombin
2. osteodystrophy
3. leukocytosis
4. dysphagia

5. karyorrhexis
6. lymphocytopenia
7. angiolith
8. hemopathology
9. angiorrhaphy
10. erythrocyte

Chapter 5

1. dolichocephalic
2. amphibious
3. preganglionic
4. intravenous
5. neurasthenia
6. anencephalia
7. lithotripsy
8. extracystic
9. electroencephalogram
10. macroscelia

Chapter 6

1. hemigastrectomy
2. celiomyalgia
3. hematemesis
4. procteurynter
5. cholecystoclysis
6. typhlatonia
7. adenemphraxis
8. amylodyspepsia
9. copremia
10. laparoscopy

Chapter 7

1. osteoarthritis
2. spondylosyndesis
3. craniodysosteosis
4. synarthrophysis
5. bursolith
6. patellar
7. arthredema
8. chondroid
9. osteosarcoma
10. tarsoptosis

Chapter 8

1. xerocheilia
2. antitussive
3. bronchorrhagia
4. pneumolithiasis
5. sinusitis
6. eupnea
7. rhinorrhagia
8. aerodermectasia
9. dyspnea
10. tracheotomy

Chapter 9

1. hematuria
2. aerourethroscopy
3. urocyanosis
4. urethremphraxis
5. nephrohypertrophy
6. pyelogram
7. pyuria
8. polyuria
9. cystoid
10. uropoiesis

Chapter 10

1. oscheoma
2. phallorrhea
3. seminuria
4. vasectomy
5. colpeurynter
6. dysmenorrhea
7. oophoropexy
8. cryptorchidism
9. exogamy
10. oviparous
11. cryptomenia
12. salpingocyesis
13. amniocentesis
14. metrorrhagia
15. aspermia
16. anorchism
17. oligomenorrhea
18. bradytocia
19. spermatoschesis
20. seminiferous

Chapter 12

1. blepharoptosis
2. corectasia
3. diplopia
4. ophthalmologist
5. mastoidotomy
6. otitis
7. hypacousia
8. symblepharosis
9. corectopia
10. dacryostenosis
11. anisocoria
12. xerophthalmia
13. otorrhea
14. intraocular
15. macrotia
16. achromatopsia
17. otosclerosis
18. aphacia
19. myringomycosis
20. phacomalacia

750
12
1500
750
9000

1750
3
5250
9000
3000
17.250